Véronique Mottier

SEXUALITY

A Very Short Introduction

OXFORD
UNIVERSITY PRESS

OXFORD

UNIVERSITY PRESS

Great Clarendon Street, Oxford OX2 6DP

Oxford University Press is a department of the University of Oxford.
It furthers the University's objective of excellence in research, scholarship,
and education by publishing worldwide in

Oxford New York

Auckland Cape Town Dar es Salaam Hong Kong Karachi
Kuala Lumpur Madrid Melbourne Mexico City Nairobi
New Delhi Shanghai Taipei Toronto

With offices in

Argentina Austria Brazil Chile Czech Republic France Greece
Guatemala Hungary Italy Japan Poland Portugal Singapore
South Korea Switzerland Thailand Turkey Ukraine Vietnam

Oxford is a registered trade mark of Oxford University Press
in the UK and in certain other countries

Published in the United States
by Oxford University Press Inc., New York

© Véronique Mottier 2008

The moral rights of the author have been asserted

Database right Oxford University Press (maker)

First published 2008

British Library Cataloguing in Publication Data

Data available

Library of Congress Cataloging in Publication Data

Mottier, Véronique.
Sexuality: a very short introduction / Véronique Mottier.
p.   cm. – (Very short introductions)
Includes bibliographical references and index.
ISBN-13: 978-0-19-929802-0
1. Sex.   2. Sex–History.   3. Women and erotica.   4. Sex–Political aspects.   I. Title.
HQ12.M68   2008
306. 709–dc22   2008000937

ISBN 978-0-19-929802-0

1 3 5 7 9 10 8 6 4 2

Typeset by SPI Publisher Services, Pondicherry, India
Printed in Great Britain by
Ashford Colour Press Ltd, Gosport, Hampshire

Sexuality: A Very Short Introduction

VERY SHORT INTRODUCTIONS are for anyone wanting a stimulating and accessible way in to a new subject. They are written by experts, and have been published in more than 25 languages worldwide.

The series began in 1995, and now represents a wide variety of topics in history, philosophy, religion, science, and the humanities. Over the next few years it will grow to a library of around 200 volumes – a Very Short Introduction to everything from ancient Egypt and Indian philosophy to conceptual art and cosmology.

Very Short Introductions available now:

For more information visit our websites
www.oup.com/uk/vsi
www.oup.com/us

Contents

Acknowledgements

Parts of this book were first developed in conjunction with my lecture series on 'Sexuality and Social Exclusion', 'Sexuality and the Dynamics of Intimacy', and 'Gender, Sexualities and the State' at the Faculty of Social and Political Sciences and the Centre for Gender Studies of the University of Cambridge between 1999 and 2008. Many thanks to students and other audiences for their probing questions and feedback. The book also draws upon some of my previous research, which was financially supported by the Swiss National Science Foundation (grants 61-66003.01 and 3346-61710.00). I thank Jesus College, Cambridge, and the Institute of Anthropology and Sociology, University of Lausanne, for institutional support.

I am deeply grateful for helpful comments and suggestions from Max Bergman, Lucy Bland, Terrell Carver, Clare Chambers, Jackie Clackson, John Cornwell, Christine Delphy, Rebecca Flemming, Peter Garnsey, Natalia Gerodetti, Anthony Giddens, Simon Goldhill, Geoff Harcourt, Wendy Harcourt, Tim Jenkins, Gerry Kearns, Duncan Kelly, Philippa Levine, Juliet Mitchell, Helen Morales, Martine Moret, Ilja Mottier, Yannis Papadaniel, Patricia Roux, Rupert Russell, Janet Soskice, Bernard Voutat, and Hans Wijngaards. I am also grateful to James Thompson, Andrea Keegan, and Marsha Filion from Oxford University

Press for suggesting and supporting this project; and to Olaf Henricson-Bell and Alyson Silverwood for copy-editing the text. It goes without saying that on such contested terrain, the views of the above are not necessarily reflected in this volume. Last but not least, many thanks to my husband James Clackson for numerous scholarly as well as other contributions.

List of illustrations

The publisher and the author apologize for any errors or omissions in the above list. If contacted they will be pleased to rectify these at the earliest opportunity.

Introduction

Sex is everywhere in the modern world. We are surrounded by
a cacophony of advice columns, celebrities, agony aunts, chat
shows, TV evangelists, therapists, women's and men's magazines,
and self-help literature which tells us how to conduct our
intimate relationships. Sexual imagery is used to sell us everyday
products such as cars or clothes, or to sell sex itself, while sex aids,
porn, and potential sex partners – real or virtual – are just one
click away on the Internet. Modernity is a world populated by
people who define themselves as gay, lesbian, straight, bisexual,
bi-curious, exhibitionists, submissives, dominatrixes, swingers
(people who engage in partner exchange), switchers (people who
change from being gay to being straight or vice versa), traders (gay
men who have sex with straight men), born-again virgins (people
who have, technically, lost their virginity but pledge to renounce
sex until marriage), acrotomophiliacs (people who are sexually
attracted to amputees), furverts (or furries – people who dress
up in animal suits and derive sexual excitement from doing so),
or feeders (people who overfeed their, generally obese, partners).
The important point here is that we draw on these categories in
order to make sense of who we are: we define ourselves in part
through our sexuality. How have we come to believe that sex
is so important to who we are? As we shall see in this volume,
this linking of 'sexuality', understood as the way in which people
experience their bodies, pleasures, and desires, with sexual

identity is in fact a modern phenomenon, which has emerged
only in the course of the 18th and 19th centuries in Europe. That
is not to say that people did not engage in sexual activities before
modernity. Rather, the way in which people made sense of their
erotic experiences was radically different from contemporary
understandings of sexuality.

Sex is a cultural object. Just as the differences between men and
women cannot be reduced to biological factors alone, but are more
adequately understood in terms of the concept of 'gender' which
takes into account the social meanings that different societies
attach to masculinity and femininity, sexuality is not a natural,
biological, universal experience. The ways in which different
cultures and different time periods have made sense of erotic
pleasures and dangers vary widely. Sexuality is shaped by social
and political forces and connects in important ways to relations
of power around class, race, and, especially, gender. Indeed, this
book will demonstrate that sex, gender, and sexuality are closely
intertwined; cultural understandings of sexuality have been
structured by normative ideas about masculinity and femininity,
in other words, 'proper' ways for men and women to behave.

Against this backdrop, this volume will explore social and
political meanings and struggles around sexuality in modernity,
primarily – though not exclusively – in the West. The main focus
will thus not be on people's concrete sexual practices, but rather
on raising sexuality as a social and political question. Chapter 1
examines historical ways of thinking about sex, focusing on ideas
developed in antiquity and Christianity, while Chapter 2 analyses
theories, controversies, and disagreements around models of
sexuality in modernity. Chapters 3, 4, and 5 further elaborate the
main theme of sexuality as a site of social and political struggle,
by focusing on challenges 'from below' in the form of feminist
critiques of sexuality (Chapter 3), the regulation of sexuality
'from above' by the state (Chapter 4), and gay politics, religious
fundamentalist mobilizations, and the future of sex (Chapter 5).

Chapter 1
Before sexuality

Male lions don't desire male lions, because lions don't do
philosophy.

ps-Lucian, c. 4th century AD

Sex in the ancient world

In Plato's *Symposium*, Aristophanes tells a story about the origins
of human beings. According to his myth, humans descend from
creatures who had spherical bodies, genitals on the outside,
four hands and feet, two faces each, and were divided into three
genders: one group had two male genitals; the second group
had two female genitals; and the third group, hermaphrodites,
had one of each. Over time, the creatures became arrogant and
uppity. To punish them, Zeus split them in two. In that state, they
clung to their other halves, dying from hunger and self-neglect
because 'they did not like to do anything apart'. Zeus took pity
on them, and invented a new plan, moving their genitals so that
they could have sexual relations with each other. Each of us is a
half of a human being, and each seeks his or her other half. Men
who are split from the hermaphrodite desire women; women who
descend from a female creature 'do not care for men, but have
female attachments'; and men who are split from a male body
prefer to pursue males, and in their boyhood 'enjoy lying with

and embracing men ... because they have the most manly nature, and ... rejoice in what is like themselves'.

Aristophanes' speech became a famous myth of origin, but what does it mean? At first sight, it seems to suggest that the ancient Greeks thought that some people desired only members of their own sex. Many classicists disagree, however, and point out that it is not for nothing that Plato has Aristophanes, the comic poet who is always coming up with the most outrageous, playfully ironic, and ultimately absurd suggestions such as a parliament of birds or women entering politics, tell this story. Certainly, for most Graeco-Romans, the idea of classifying people according to the gender of the person they have sex with would have seemed downright bizarre. Antiquity was not a culture of sexual libertarianism. Sexual morality was highly regulated by moral and legal rules. However, moral preoccupations centred on sexual practices, not on the subject of desire. The ancients did not make sense of themselves in terms of sexual identities, whereas the policing of gender identity was of central importance to them, as we shall see. Consider the contrast with the ways in which modern subjects make sense of their sexual experiences. Categories such as heterosexual and homosexual are a central source upon which we draw in order to make sense of our own sexuality. It is in this sense that the classical world has been described as a world 'before sexuality' by historians such as Michel Foucault, Paul Veyne, David Halperin, or John Winkler. The ways in which sex was conceptualized and the cultural meanings that were attached to it were radically different from today.

Sexual culture was far from homogeneous across the ancient world. Substantial regional and historical variations existed, which cannot be done justice to in the format of the present short introduction. In this section, therefore, we will concentrate primarily on classical Athens and Rome. Taking a closer look at the ways in which ancient Athenians and Romans made sense of sex will provide a useful backdrop and contrast against which

4

we can draw out critical questions about sex in the modern world.

Classical Athenian sexual culture must be located in its social and political context. Greek society was based on the political and social rule of a small elite of adult male citizens; citizen women and children occupied a socially subordinate position and had no political rights, and immigrants and slaves had no citizenship status. More precisely, Athenian women had the status of minors and were always under legal guardianship of a male relative. Reflecting the social power of male citizens, sexual culture was organized around male pleasure. The ancients adopted a phallocentric notion of sex, defined exclusively as penetration. While kisses, caresses, and forms of touching other than penetration were considered expressions of love, they were not considered part of the sexual domain. Sex was thus not construed in relational terms, as a shared experience reflecting emotional intimacy, but as something – penetration – done to someone else. The physical pleasure, or indeed collaboration, of the partner was broadly considered to be irrelevant. Men were encouraged to use penetrative sex for domination and control of the submissive partner. Sex reflected social and political relations of power, since men performed their social status as citizens in the arenas of war, politics, and sex.

Sexual culture was closely intertwined with notions of sex and gender. Medical knowledge of the time saw bodies as fragile, consisting of liquids in a precarious balance affected by age, diet, and lifestyle. Ageing and, ultimately, death was understood as a process of cooling and drying out of the body. Consequently, cultural preoccupations emerged with diet and other ways of maintaining a healthy equilibrium of fluids within the body. Following Galen, the 2nd-century AD Roman author of medical treatises, gender was similarly understood as a fluid state. Men were seen as active, hot, and strong; women as passive, weak, damp, and cold, losing body heat and vital energy through leakage such as menstruation, and robbing men of their heat and energy through sex. Sex itself was conceptualized as involving heating of the body. Aesthetically, the Greeks seem to have had a preference for male bodies with puny penises, with the added benefit that they were less at risk in war.

As the historian Thomas Laqueur has pointed out, the classical model of gender involved a 'one-sex model': since gender was understood as fluid, men risked becoming more feminized if they lost heat, while women could become more like men if their bodies heated up. The psychological consequence of such beliefs was that gender did not appear as a stable, biological characteristic, but as an identity that was potentially under threat. Men risked feminization when losing vital body heat, as they might during excessive amounts of sexual intercourse with cold female bodies and loss of liquids through ejaculation. While sex was thought necessary for good health, too much of it was thus considered dangerous for men. In contrast, women's cold, moist bodies needed male sexual heat to compensate for their lack of vitality. Even more crucially, women needed the liquidity of seed in order to keep the womb stable (which the Hippocratic school of medicine believed to be free-floating), so that it didn't wander off in search of moisture elsewhere in the woman's body and end up suffocating her.

Such medical beliefs were reflected in the view held by the ancient Graeco-Romans that all women were by nature oversexed, as echoed in the myth of Tiresias, which is best known in the version in Ovid's *Metamorphoses*. Ovid tells the story of the man Tiresias who was, for seven years, transformed into a woman by the gods, before reverting back to his male body. Having experienced sex both as a man and as a woman, Tiresias was later asked to settle a dispute between the god Zeus and his wife Hera as to whether it is men or women whose sexual pleasure is more intense. When he declared that it was women, Hera struck him blind in retaliation for having given away this female secret.

Considered inferior creatures to men, women were seen as lacking the male capacity for sexual self-control. Female sexuality was therefore dangerous, since women's sexual voracity could exhaust men or, worse, turn them into women. In a society where the social and civic status of women was extremely low, male anxieties centred on the need to stabilize masculinity by establishing and policing gender boundaries. Male gender identity was fragile, since masculinity was not founded on the possession of a male body (because the body was seen as unstable and at risk of slipping into femininity), but on the aggressive performance of masculinity in everyday life, including in the sphere of sexual interactions. In defending one's masculinity against potential attacks, male sexual performance, rather than male sexual desire, was central. Flagging of male lust was consequently seen as a humiliating failure of masculinity, and was a frequent source of comedy in novels and plays. In one of the best-known passages on male sexual misfortune in classical literature, the hero of Petronius's Roman novel *Satyricon*, Encolpius, attempts to have sex with the beautiful Circe, who has told him he must give up his 16-year-old boyfriend Giton for her, when disaster strikes:

> Three times I whip the dreadful weapon out,
> And three times softer than a Brussels sprout
> I quail, in those dire straits my manhood blunted,
> No longer up to what just now I wanted.

As suggested by the medical author Priscianus, erotic imagery was thought to be a cure for declining virility: 'Let the patient be surrounded by beautiful girls or boys; also give him books to read, which stimulate lust and in which love-stories are insinuatingly treated.' Failing that, dancing girls, or various aphrodisiac stimulants, catalogued at great length by Pliny the Elder in his *Natural History*, were recommended. More generally, sexual imagery, and especially images of the erect phallus, a symbol of male power used to ward off evil, was present everywhere in everyday life in the ancient world.

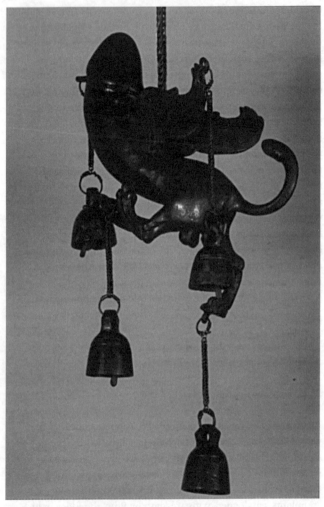

1. Winged phallus from Pompeii, probably used for home decoration, 1st century AD

Archaeological evidence suggests that frescoes, wall-paintings, graffiti, and sculptures of the erect phallus and other sexual and fertility imagery would adorn the gardens and homes of wealthy households, as well as everyday household objects such as wind-chimes or pottery. Dildos and other sexual aids are frequently mentioned in ancient literature and depicted on pottery, while didactic sex manuals were popular, as were more general advice books such as the *Ars Amatoria* by the Roman poet Ovid which contained three books of advice to the prospective lover, followed by his *Remedia Amoris* which proffered handy tips to those suffering from heartbreak.

Normative ideas of masculinity valued aggressive, dominant behaviour, both in public speaking and in other areas of life, including sexual activity. Masculinity was identified with the active, penetrative sexual role. Sexual desire was seen as normal or deviant in relation to the extent to which it transgressed normative gender roles. Specific practices such as sodomy or masturbation did not give rise to moral anxieties in classical sexual culture. Questions of sexual etiquette centred instead on penetration. Penetration symbolized male as well as social status, but it mattered little whether the penetrated was a woman or a boy. What did matter was who penetrated whom. Penetration was seen as active, submission to penetration as passive. It was considered unnatural and demeaning for a free-born man to desire to be penetrated, since that would reduce him to the socially inferior role of a woman or slave. 'Proper' objects of penetration were women, boys, foreigners, and slaves, all categories of people who did not enjoy the same political or social citizenship rights as the free Athenian male citizens. Social status was negotiated around the active/passive distinction, not on the basis of heterosexual/homosexual categorization, which only emerged much later in history.

Rules governing sex were thus structured by the norms of political citizenship. As the classicist David Halperin puts it: 'Citizenship, for free Athenian men, was a sexual and gendered concept as well as a political and social one', and antiquity promoted an 'ethos of penetration and domination' which conflated the sexual order with the political and the social order. Antiquity thus did not make a clear distinction between the public, political sphere and the private, sexual sphere. Accusations of sexual impropriety were commonly used weapons against political opponents. This widespread sexual abuse in public discourse could be very explicit, and could have important consequences for the abused, including loss of citizenship. Within the hierarchy of sexual acts, the most demeaning was the accusation of cunnilingus, closely followed by that of fellatio since being penetrated in the mouth by a penis was considered degrading for either man or woman (and therefore best practised with prostitutes or slaves). People from the island of Lesbos had the reputation of engaging in particularly depraved sexual activities. It is thus that for the ancient Greeks, the verb 'lesbiazein' meant 'act like a lesbian', or more particularly, 'fellate', with no gender specificity except for the recipient.

Relationships between men were socially acceptable, common, and widely reflected in the literature, art, and philosophy of the time. Attitudes on male-to-male sex were not homogeneous, however, and disputes on whether desire for young men or for women was superior abounded. Some argued that love for men was superior to that for women, since love between equals was preferable to that for inferior creatures. As the *Erotes*, an ancient Greek dialogue of uncertain authorship on the respective advantages of love for men and for women, puts it:

> Marriage is a remedy devised by the necessity of procreation, but male love alone must rule the heart of a philosopher.

The text goes on to argue that sex with women serves the natural need for procreation, but that once such basic needs are fulfilled and society develops to a higher stage, men would naturally want to pursue forms of gratification which were all the more culturally superior for their lack of naturalness:

> Just because commerce with women has an older pedigree than that with boys, do not disdain the latter. Let's remember that the very first discoveries were prompted by need, but those which arose from progress are only the better for it, and worthier of our esteem.

Greek poetry promoted the idea that it was best to have armies composed of male lovers since warriors would fight hardest and be bravest in order to save and impress their lovers – an argument also put forward in Plato's *Symposium*. Plato himself, however, was among those who expressed discomfort about male-to-male sex. Most criticism centred on men who enjoyed the passive, submissive role. Such men were seen as soft and effeminate, who were really women in male bodies. By their transgression of the normative models of gender, effeminate, submissive males who voluntarily adopted the socially inferior position of women by offering their bodies to be penetrated were seen as unnatural, and a shocking threat to the social order, in the same way as women who adopted the male role (called *tribades*).

Given the importance of the penetrative role for male social and political status, relationships between adult men were a source of great anxiety, since one of the partners would have to adopt the submissive role. Relationships with boys solved this problem to some degree, since adolescent men achieved citizenship status only when reaching adult age. Classical culture had a sexual revulsion towards the idea of hair growing on a young man's cheeks or thighs. Boys were considered sexually desirable from the start of puberty until late adolescence, but stopped being so at the appearance of the beard and pubic hair. Athenians considered love affairs between adult and adolescent males as natural and honourable, on condition that sexual etiquette was respected.

The term used to describe the sexual pursuit of adolescent males by adult males was 'paederastia'. In stark contrast to modern attitudes towards sex between teachers and students, paederastia was usually conceptualized as a pedagogic and erotic mentoring relationship between an adult male, the 'erastes' (lover), and a young, passive 'pais' (boy) called the 'eromenos' (beloved), usually between 12 and 17–20 years old (though professional teachers and trainers, often former slaves, were not allowed to seduce their students, nor were slaves allowed to seduce young free-born males). Often presented as a normal part of the education of a young man, paederastia institutionalized a relationship in which the mentor instructed the boy in philosophical matters and general knowledge, and prepared him for his citizenship role.

Despite general social acceptance of paederastic relationships, the fact that free-born boys were future citizens entailed a certain degree of moral preoccupation about social status. It was therefore crucial to observe sexual etiquette in this area. In particular, boys were not expected to experience sexual desire in the paederastic relationship. If they conceded sexual favours to the older man, this was expected to be out of 'philia' – friendship, respect, and affection for the suitor. It was thought proper that boys should submit only after a respectably long and sometimes expensive courtship. Deriving sexual pleasure from male-to-male sex could open the boy up to accusations of 'feminine' shamelessness and 'less than male behaviour' (given women's supposedly voracious appetite for sexual pleasure).

Little material exists on sex between women, and historians of sex in antiquity such as Halperin or Foucault focus almost exclusively on male-to-male sex. The work of the 7th-century BC poet Sappho, born on Lesbos, is one of the rare examples of sources describing intense infatuations and love between women, though little of it survives. Male views of female-to-female sex in antiquity usually mention such practices in disapproving, contemptuous terms or, alternatively, reflect voyeuristic interest. They habitually imagine women who have sex with women as having an enlarged clitoris similar to a penis, or as adopting the male penetrative role with the aid of strap-on penises.

Although male-to-male sex has been the most intensely debated feature of classical sexual culture, it was part of a much wider landscape of male sexual options, including commercial sex and marriage. Legitimate marriage, and sex within it, was expected of every citizen whether male or female, and was a fundamental obligation to society. Respectable women were out of bounds for sexual liaisons except in marriage, which formed the limits of their sexual horizons. Adultery, defined as sexual activity involving a married woman (with the marital status of the adulterer irrelevant), was the paradigmatic ancient sex crime, and an obsession in much ancient literature. Whereas most sexual misbehaviour in the ancient world was sanctioned informally, through public censure and social dishonour, adultery could lead to complex legal consequences. Seduction of a free Athenian woman was a crime which was generally deemed more serious than rape, because a secret liaison meant that a man could not be sure of the lineage of his children, whereas in the case of rape any offspring could be identified and killed. Rape was thus primarily seen as a crime against the husband, father, or male guardian of the woman rather than against herself, and as a threat to public order due to the risk of revenge from the aggrieved male party (who was legally allowed to put the perpetrator of any adultery – whether consensual or the result of rape – to death if caught in the act). The Roman *lex Iulia* on adultery, introduced by the emperor Augustus in 17 BC, redefined adultery from being a family matter to an offence whose punishment – exile or death – was enshrined in law, and in which the whole of society had a stake. Indeed, if a husband or father failed to bring a prosecution within a certain time frame, any concerned citizen could do so.

Although spending money on dancing girls, 'nightwalkers', and other categories of prostitutes was seen as a regrettable sign of a lack of self-control, it was nevertheless considered a more respectable and certainly less risky alternative for men to illegal sex with free women. Commercial sex was freely available across the ancient world. In many Greek and Roman cities, prostitutes paid tax and thus made significant contributions to local economies. Clients were exclusively men, but prostitutes could be women as well as young and adolescent men (most often ex-slaves and other non-citizens). Sexual assignments seem to have been conducted openly both in brothels and in public spaces such as parks and cemeteries, and archaeological remains of sandals which left an imprint on the ground with the words 'follow me' illustrate forms of soliciting by streetwalkers. Men could also buy a sex slave for exclusive relations, or divide the cost among friends. For wealthy men, the use of sophisticated courtesans (*hetairai*) was an additional and socially acceptable option. As the prominent 4th-century BC Greek statesman Demosthenes put it: 'we have *hetairai* for delectation, concubines for the daily servicing of our bodies, and wives to bear legitimate offspring and to be faithful protectors of the households'. Successful courtesans – most often former slaves and immigrants – enjoyed a much greater degree of autonomy than women from citizen families, and some of them achieved great wealth and public stature.

Sexual access to the submissive bodies of women or male adolescents by sexually assertive men was of central importance for the political order of classical Athens. Classical Greeks credited Solon, the founding father of Athenian democracy, with the democratization of access to sex slaves through the establishment of public brothels in which the price of prostitutes was kept affordable for any citizen, although the factual correctness of this account is disputed. As David Halperin points out, the importance of this story lies in the link it makes between prostitution and political democracy: all male citizens, rich or poor, should be able to afford access to sexual pleasure. The provision of cheap prostitutes allowed free men whose poverty risked putting them in a socially subordinate, and therefore feminized, position to maintain their social dominance through sexual domination. Historical evidence, such as pricing information found on the walls of brothels in Pompeii, suggests that prostitutes were indeed generally cheap in the ancient world (with services in the lower price range comparable to the cost of a loaf of bread), though prices varied considerably across time and place.

The problematization of male prostitution illustrates the intricate link between sex, gender, and politics in antiquity; although male prostitution was not illegal, free men who prostituted themselves were seen to lower themselves to the level of women, immigrants, and slaves by accepting the role of sexual object. Any male Athenian who had engaged in prostitution in his youth consequently forfeited his civil and political citizenship rights.

In addition to citizenship, sex in the ancient world was also intertwined with religious practice. Some public holidays, such as an annual religious festival in Canopus in Roman Egypt, were celebrated specifically by sex, dancing, singing, and other rituals. No convincing evidence exists of temple prostitution in ancient Greece or Rome, in contrast to the ancient Near East, where the practice of sacred slave-prostitutes serving visitors was widespread; but prostitutes did have their own religious festivals in Rome, and more generally attended religious festivals either as worshippers or to work the crowds.

However, it is important to remember that Rome and Athens did not form a single homogeneous, unitary culture. Whereas Roman sexual ethics were quite similar to those of classical Greece, the most marked difference was that sodomy was much more problematic within Roman culture, and paederastic relationships (and their supposed educational advantages) were not generally idealized. Relations with free-born men and boys were legally prohibited in Roman morality laws such as the *lex Iulia*, though it was legal for a free man to have sex with male prostitutes, slaves, or foreign young men (as long as he performed the active role), or to frequent brothels. Such laws were periodically re-enacted in the Empire to demonstrate the respective emperors' concern for public morality; however, they were rarely enforced. Reflecting Greek cultural influence, revered Roman poets such as Catullus, Ovid, Horace, and Virgil wrote of love affairs between men, and one of Tibullus' poems described his heartbreak at having been left for a woman by his young male lover Marathus.

The civic status of women was higher in Imperial Rome than in Athens, where women's names were not allowed to be mentioned in public until after their death. Roman women (at least, those of the propertied class) showed greater independence than women in classical Athens. For example, although in law Roman women had to have guardians, in practice this was gradually phased out, and upper-class women could own and have control over property (after the death of their father). Sexual misbehaviour, especially by women, came to stand for wider anxieties over alleged corruption and moral decline in the Roman context. Sexual transgressions, such as adultery or sex with slaves, by upper-class women were declared criminal offences in the Roman morality laws (though again, rarely subject to actual legal prosecution), and literary material of the time reflects male anxieties about such female behaviour.

The historian and social theorist Michel Foucault has argued that Graeco-Roman rules of sexual conduct need to be located in the context of a wider set of concerns with how to be a good citizen, which included prescriptions on diet, exercise, and relations with subordinates such as wives and slaves more generally. He also pointed out that, in comparison, cultural anxieties over food were much more important than those over sex in Greek and Roman culture. Indeed, the ancient world, where everyday life was for many a struggle for survival, was 'obsessed with food', in the words of ancient historian Peter Garnsey. Preoccupations with diet and regime intensified among the Romans. In a context where the social and political power of upper-class male citizens knew few bounds and cultural anxieties about moral decline were rife, Stoic philosophers such as Seneca developed an ethos of self-control that was intended to demonstrate male elites' mastery over their appetites while also avoiding the supposed ill effects of food, drink, or sex binges. As Seneca put it: 'Morality has collapsed, perversity reigns, humanity is in decay, crime is spreading.' However, as he added in his letter to his friend Lucilius:

> You are wrong, Lucilius, if you think that luxury, contempt for morality and other vices are merely vices of our time: vices for which everyone reproves his own age. They are the defects of humankind, not of the times. No era has ever been free from blame.

To counter such propensity for hedonism, an ethos of self-mastery was presented as a morally pleasing alternative, part of an aesthetics of existence which made one's life beautiful. Leading a virtuous life meant self-imposed moderation and balance 'in all things'. Sexual self-restraint was part of this wider ethos focused on the paterfamilias, to whom any member of the household – not just his wife – was potentially sexually available.

Drawing on Hippocratic medicine, Plato, and Aristotle, Roman physicians such as Galen further emphasized the dangers of 'excess' and the benefits of nutritional and sexual frugality. Regarding sexual ethics, whereas sexual intercourse in moderation was considered necessary for health reasons, sexual excesses should be avoided since they were thought to result in feebleness, impotence, and wasting diseases for men. The famous scholar Pliny the Elder thus pointed approvingly at the example of elephants in his *Natural History*, since 'their intercourse takes place only every second year, and for five days only, and no more; on the sixth day they plunge into a river, before doing which they will not rejoin the herd'. But the concept of self-mastery also had political relevance. Eros, the force of love and desire, was feared as being potentially disruptive of the social and political order. Tyrants were typically accused of uncontrollable sexual self-indulgence, and the management of personal appetites was thus seen as essential for the survival of democratic rule, as Michel Foucault has pointed out. In the words of the ancient historian James Davidson: 'the Greeks ... felt a civic responsibility to manage all appetites, to train themselves to deal with them, without trying to conquer them absolutely'. By the 5th century AD, a culture of self-mastery had thus established itself among elites. This culture valued sexual moderation and, intertwined with early Christian influences, forms of sexual renunciation. However, despite some continuities between classical and Christian ethics, the rise of Christianity would radically transform the social and political meanings attached to sex.

Christianity and the corruptions of the flesh

Early Christianity incorporated some of the ideas on self-mastery already present in Late Antiquity, but reworked them to formulate a radically new sexual ethics. Whereas in Late Antiquity, sexual renunciation was valued as part of a male ethics of self-mastery, by the 5th century AD, Christian ideals promoted virginity and sexual abstinence for men as well as women. In the context of a shift in political power towards church authorities, sexual desire came to be blamed for binding humans to their worldly obligations to spouse or children. It prevented them from concentrating on spirituality in furtherance of the coming of the kingdom of heaven, and preparation for the afterlife. Christian hostility towards sex reflects this wider religious project of freeing humans from their worldly ties and desires. Celibacy and purity came to be valorized, whereas sex and desire became policed.

A key influence in this development was Augustine (354–430 AD), one of the founding fathers of Western Christianity, whose gloomy teachings developed the influential doctrine of 'original sin' which presented sex as the cause of the expulsion of Adam and Eve from the Garden of Eden narrated in Genesis. Augustine declared that sexual intercourse in paradise would have taken the form of 'a gentle falling asleep in the partner's arms' had Adam and Eve not fallen prey to carnal desire, and that 'lustful sex is the enemy of God'. In contrast to the classical age, for Augustine sex was not produced by the heating of the body, but by 'concupiscence' – sinful desire. Man's fall from grace expressed the victory of the 'corruptions of the flesh' over moral will power, and intercourse was tainted by original sin. Consequently, Augustine promoted sexual abstinence even though he himself had not found the struggle against 'the filth of concupiscence' easy, as reflected in his autobiographical work *Confessions*, in which he famously described himself as a youth praying to God to 'give me chastity and continence, only not yet'.

Christian ethics therefore developed a notable hostility towards sex and, more generally, towards carnal desire, which it saw as an obstacle to spiritual salvation, chaining humans to their animal lusts. The taint of sin was thought to pollute humans from the moment of birth. As Calvin put it, a newborn baby is 'a seedbed of sin and therefore cannot but be odious and abominable to God'. Whereas for the ancient Greeks and Romans, the erect phallus was a symbol of power, for Augustine it incarnated man's enslavement to concupiscence. Women were presented as even greater 'slaves to lust … worse than beasts', in the words of Origen, a Greek theologian of the 3rd century AD.

Christian attitudes towards marriage were ambivalent. Following Jesus's cue that 'if anyone comes to me and does not hate his father and mother, his wife and children, his brothers and sisters – yes, even his own life – he cannot be my disciple' (Luke 14: 26), early Christians saw families fundamentally as obstacles to religious devotion. Marriage was all the more viewed with suspicion due to the dangers of the temptations of the flesh, which reflected the works of the devil. As Pope Innocent III formulated this dilemma in the 13th century: 'everyone knows that intercourse, even between married persons, is never performed without the itch of the flesh, the heat of passion and the stench of lust'. The Protestant theologian Martin Luther shared this distaste for marital intercourse, declaring that 'had God consulted me in the matter, I would have advised him to continue the generation of the species by fashioning them out of clay'. However, Church fathers recognized that the majority of believers were unlikely to adopt the Christian ideal of the celibate life. Marriage was therefore seen as an acceptable compromise with the material world, and praised as a building block for society by theologians such as Paul who argued that spouses owed each other the 'marriage debt' of sexual intercourse as long as procreative motivations were their main purpose, and they observed monogamy and fidelity. This put a greater onus on the procreative aspects of marriage than in the ancient world, where adoption of children or adults had constituted a socially acceptable alternative to the production of heirs through reproduction. Sexual consummation of the marriage became consequently of crucial importance in the Christian world, and non-consummation was declared legitimate ground for divorce in Gratian's textbook of canon law (1140 AD). However, Church authorities generally viewed requests for dissolution of marriage with suspicion, since unscrupulous spouses might use false claims of impotence as a way of freeing themselves of a marriage. For this reason, various regions, including England, introduced the examination of husbands by 'honest women' in the service of Church courts. In his book *Impotence: A Cultural History* the historian Angus McLaren reports an account of such an examination provided to the courts of York and Canterbury in the 15th century:

> The same witness exposed her naked breasts, and with her hands warmed at the said fire, she hid and rubbed the penis and testicles of the said John. And she embraced and frequently kissed the same John, and stirred him up in so far as she could to show his virility and potency, admonishing him that for shame he should

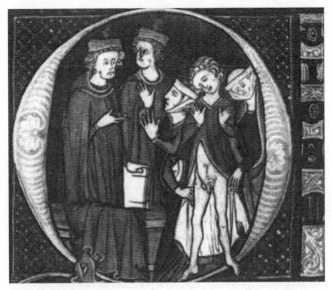

2. Medieval examination to demonstrate impotence, then regarded as legitimate grounds to terminate a marriage contract

then and there prove himself a man. And she says, examined and diligently questioned, that the whole time aforesaid, the said penis was scarcely three inches long, … remaining without any increase or decrease.

On the grounds that 'to many, total abstinence is easier than perfect moderation', as Augustine put it, Christian marriage was presented as second-best to celibacy and other ascetic practices. Some early Church fathers such as Origen were said to take the fight against spiritual pollution from lustful desires so far as to have castrated themselves. Although never very popular with the wider population, by the 4th century self-castration as an expression of Christian chastity had sufficiently alarmed Church authorities for them to condemn the practice in various Church regulations and to declare it heretic. Others, such as the Desert

Fathers Anthony and Jerome in the 3rd and 4th centuries, retreated into the Egyptian desert, a practice of withdrawal from the material world which later became institutionalized in the form of monasteries.

Given the emphasis on reproductive sex within marriage and the disapproval of other lustful sexual practices, same-sex relationships between women were consistently condemned and suppressed by Church authorities, though rarely subject to legal prosecution. Church attitudes towards male same-sex relationships seem to have been more contradictory. Although the extent to which relationships between men were tolerated is a topic of controversy among historians, the medieval historian John Boswell records examples of same-sex unions between men that seem to have been sanctioned by religious ceremonies, arguing that such partnerships were 'commonplace' in early medieval Byzantine society and that it was only from the 14th century onwards that such practices were repressed by the Catholic Church. It is certainly the case that practices of repression of male-to-male sex varied widely across different regions and time periods. Christian ethics condemned sodomy as a sinful act against nature, but until the 18th century sodomy remained a catch-all term which included a variety of 'unnatural' (in the sense of non-procreative) practices performed by men or by women such as bestiality, masturbation, anal and oral sex, sex between two men or two women, or intercourse between a man and a woman with the aim of avoiding conception.

Renaissance Florence had a reputation for being a sinful city where the vice of sodomy flourished, and in 1432, the city created the Office of the Night, a magistracy whose sole purpose was the prosecution of sodomy. The historian Michael Rocke describes how during a period of 70 years, 17,000 men (from a total of 40,000 inhabitants) were investigated at least once for sodomy. His legal evidence reveals both that the majority of male inhabitants of Florence seemed to have engaged in such

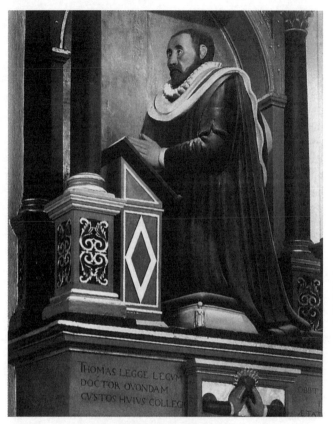

3. A memorial at Caius College, Cambridge, dated 1619. It commemorates the Master of the College, Gostlin, and his male friend Dr Legge. Below the image of the flaming heart, the inscription says: 'Love joined them living. So may the earth join them in their burial. Oh Legge, Gostlin's heart you still have with you'

practices, and that their punishment consisted in most cases of light fines. In contrast, in many other medieval and Renaissance cities across Europe such as Augsburg, Venice, or Geneva under Calvin, religious and secular authorities enforced more drastic punishments for sodomy, ranging from imprisonment and castration to beheadings, starvation, and burning at the stake. Prosecution of sodomy intensified in the 18th century, when it also shifted meaning to refer solely to sexual acts between men.

Christianity took over 1,000 years to firmly establish itself in Europe, and many different sects persisted on the fringes of the Church both during and after this period of consolidation of religious and political power. Not all of these shared the same emphasis on sexual asceticism. Groups such as the 2nd-century Egyptian Gnostic sect the Carpocratians, for example, were said to believe that in order to leave the material world, human souls had first to go through every possible earthly experience, and they were consequently notorious for their sexual libertinism, which was said to include wife-sharing and public nudity.

More generally, it should of course be remembered that the spread of Christian values did not necessarily mean that populations lived their lives in ways approved of by the Church. Christianity produced, however, a highly influential normative model of sex, which elevated virginity and celibacy as the highest spiritual ideal and a means of freeing oneself from worldly obligations, in contrast to, for example, Judaism which disapproved of abstinence as an obvious impediment against God's directive to 'be fruitful and multiply'. The idealization of sexual abstinence, worldly renunciation, or procreative sex and fidelity within marriage gave new cultural meanings to sex as the primary site of the work of Satan, and therefore as something that needed to be feared and avoided. Whereas most classical medical knowledge considered lack of sex as damaging to health, the Christian idealization of virginity and abstinence promoted a sexual order in which non-sex was presented as the highest spiritual ideal.

Chapter 2
The invention of sexuality

Careful observation among the ladies of large cities soon convinces one that homosexuality is by no means a rarity. Uranism may nearly always be suspected in females wearing their hair short, or who dress in the fashion of men, or pursue the sports and pastimes of their male acquaintances; (...) The female urning may chiefly be found in the haunts of boys. (...) Love for arts finds a substitute in the pursuits of the sciences. At times smoking and drinking are cultivated even with passion. Perfumes and sweetmeats are disdained.

Richard von Krafft-Ebing, *Psychopathia Sexualis* (1886)

The science of sex

In giving sex a special status by declaring it to be the original sin, Christianity placed sex firmly at the centre of Christian morality. The historian and social theorist Michel Foucault's *The History of Sexuality* famously pointed out the irony of Christian ethics defining sex simultaneously as something shameful, which should not be spoken about, and as the sin 'par excellence', which must be traced not just in its actual manifestations, but also in the mind's deepest-hidden desires. Through the evolution of procedures such as Catholic confession and the rigorous examination of one's own conscience fostered by the Reformation, Christianity in fact created institutional mechanisms for incessant reflection upon sex, encouraging the 'confession' of personal sexual 'truths'. At the same time as Christian moral devaluation of sex asserted itself, writers such as Casanova, Sade, Wilkes, and the author of the anonymously published Victorian text *My Secret Life*, celebrated their libertine experiences in explicit detail, an apparent contradiction which seems less so when viewed as part of the same trend towards the public narration of sexual truths initiated by the Christian confessional model. In modern times, such confessional models spread to other areas of social life such as family, relationships, medicine, therapy, criminal justice, education, and the media, all settings where we are encouraged to communicate our deepest thoughts and desires. As Foucault puts it, 'we have since become a singularly confessing society'.

Christian ethics came under attack from the Enlightenment crusade against religious dogma. A culture of sexual libertinism developed in Europe, most notably from the 17th century onwards, at first within the aristocratic elites, among whom the use of condoms, made from sheep intestines, and dildos became at the same time more widespread. From the 1850s, rubber condoms became available, although they seem to have been primarily used for protecting men against venereal disease from sex with prostitutes, and remained too expensive for the working classes. Although the subject of Church disapproval, abortion had traditionally been judged acceptable across much of Europe if carried out before the moment of 'quickening', when the woman started to be able to feel the fœtus, around the fourth month of pregnancy. Methods for aborting were publicly advertised in the 19th-century press, and the abortion industry was thriving until, in the course of that century, it started to be regulated and criminalized in most European countries.

Cultural anxieties about sex intensified in response to the rapid social and political changes brought about by industrial modernization. The linked processes of industrialization (the development of modern, mechanized methods of production), urbanization (the resulting increase in the proportion of the population living in urban centres), and secularization (the decreasing importance of religious beliefs in modern society) created large urban masses in which atomized individuals were less exposed than ever before to the social and religious control of traditional pre-modern communities. As the literary critic Steven Marcus has pointed out, the 19th century thus combined a thriving, and mostly urban, underworld of prostitution, dance halls, and a dramatic increase in the availability of pornographic material, partly driven by the development of modern print technologies, with public prudery and sexual repression. Against this backdrop, collective concerns about the decline in public and private morality that supposedly resulted from the impact of modernity intensified. Moral reform groups depicted sexual libertinism as a danger to the social order and to religion, while an extensive medical and advice literature warned of the dangers of sex and of sexually transmissible diseases to personal health.

Western culture developed in particular an obsessive interest in masturbation or 'the sin of Onan', drawing on its biblical reference. Concerns were initially triggered by an anonymously published, best-selling pamphlet that appeared in London in the early years of the Enlightenment (some time around 1712) with the title *Onania; or, the Heinous Sin of Self Pollution, and all its Frightful Consequences, in both SEXES considered, with Spiritual and Physical Advice to those who have already injured themselves by this abominable Practice*. Its author claimed that, while he initially thought that spiritual guidance would do the trick of dissuading people from this 'filthy commerce with oneself', he came to realize the superiority of a medical cure consisting of a 'strengthening tincture' and 'prolific powder', which he also happened to invent and sell at a rather hefty price. Despite its quackish nature, this text is significant in that it transforms the religious understanding of masturbation as a problem of moral weakness into a medical problem caused by ignorance of the dire consequences of 'self-abuse' on personal health, as the historian

Thomas Laqueur points out in his book *Solitary Sex: A Cultural History of Masturbation* (2003). The topic was subsequently, and avidly, taken up by key representatives of the Enlightenment. The eminent 18th-century Swiss physician Samuel Tissot produced a widely read work, *Onanism*, in 1760 which influenced the inclusion of the topic of masturbation in Diderot's *Encyclopédie*, the Enlightenment's scientific work par excellence. Voltaire saw an opportunity in Tissot's medicalization of masturbation for further attack on the clergy, whose unnatural abstinence made them, Voltaire argued, particularly prone to such unhealthy solitary pleasure, while Rousseau's work on the education of the young, *Émile* (1762), equally warned against its dire consequences.

Masturbation was held responsible for a wide range of long-term medical problems including mental exhaustion, blurred vision, defective memory, blindness, rheumatism, gout, madness, gonorrhoea, epilepsy, impotence, and various sexual deviances. By the mid-19th century, medical science invented the condition of 'spermatorrhoea' whose purported symptoms consisted of nervous debility and a general wasting of the faculties resulting from 'excessive' loss of semen due to masturbation. An anti-masturbation commerce developed which proposed cures ranging from rest, mountain walks, health spas, vigorous exercise, and cold baths to chastity belts and complex electrical devices intended to discourage masturbation by delivering electric shocks upon the perpetrators.

Female masturbation was seen as particularly deviant against the backdrop of normative ideas of female sexuality that portrayed women as less subject to 'animal passions' than men. In addition, women's physical constitutions were thought to be weaker than those of men. Masturbation was consequently considered even more dangerous to women's health, and drastic treatments could comprise surgical interventions including clitoridectomy (the removal of part or most of the female genitalia). More generally, not only grown women but also young persons (of both sexes)

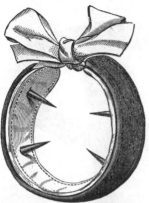

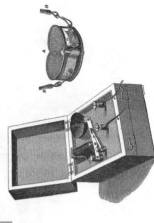

FOUR-POINTED URETHRAL RING.

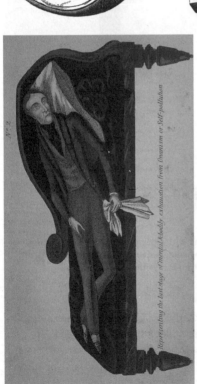

N.º 2

Representing the last stage of mental & bodily exhaustion from Onanism or Self-pollution

4. Victorian anti-masturbation devices: a penis ring; a machine delivering electric shocks to the perpetrator; and a warning of the physical and mental consequences of masturbation, from 1845

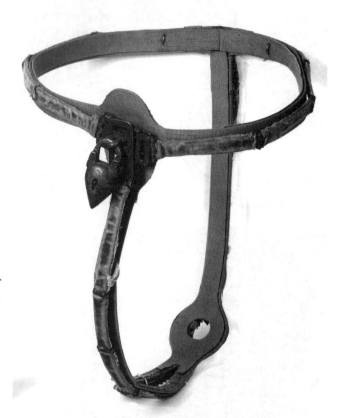

5. A chastity belt for women, with padlock, from the 16th century. Victorian chastity belts were modelled on these types of devices, but aimed to prevent masturbation rather than infidelity

were thought to be particularly prone to this dangerous practice. This reflected the wider assumption that children, being less cultured and therefore closer to nature than adults, were sexual beings with appetites that needed to be kept in check by civilizing norms – a sexualized understanding of childhood that Freud would radicalize by further arguing for the fundamentally sexual nature of children (see pp. 46–7).

Whereas in pre-industrial European societies, sexual practices were primarily subjected to moral and religious problematization and categorized in relation to sin, the social transformations brought about by modernity from the late 18th century onwards, and the Enlightenment-inspired march away from religious obscurantism towards the twin deities of science and rationality, led to new ways of thinking about sex which turned it into an object of scientific research. Modern understandings of sexuality can be traced back to the birth of the science of sex ('sexology') around the turn of the 20th century. Sex became an object of scientific study in its own right, particularly in the context of medicine and the social sciences. Darwinian theory having had a major influence on the emerging social sciences, Darwin's view of sexual selection as the key to evolution also became a major impetus for the development of modern sexual science. Through the concept of sexual selection, scientific investigations were, from their beginnings, concerned with questions of heredity, degeneracy, and race. A second major impetus for sex research was the growing concern with public health, in particular with prostitution, personal hygiene, and venereal disease. Sex research became closely intertwined with growing state intervention in sexual matters. It reflected the social and political concerns of the time, as well as its social hierarchies, which were heavily structured by class and gender.

Against this backdrop, sexuality was invented. The term 'sexuality', in its contemporary meaning of 'possession of sexual powers, or capability of sexual feelings', first entered the English language in 1879 according to the Oxford English Dictionary. The first comparable occurrence in French is attributed to the somewhat obscure novelist Péladan, who wrote of the 'animal drunkenness of sexuality' ('l'ivresse animale de la sexualité') in his erotic novel *Le vice suprême*, published in 1884. The new concept of sexuality located sex, as an area of scientific study as well as of subjective experience, firmly in the realm of nature and biology. Sexology replaced the undifferentiated religious category of sin with the medical categories of physical and mental disease and degeneracy. In the process, it radically transformed the social meanings of sex. As the sociologist Jeffrey Weeks puts it:

> Sexology was simultaneously constituting and exploring a new continent of knowledge, assigning thereby a new significance to the 'sexual'.

Biological models of sexuality dominated sexual science throughout the 19th and 20th centuries. They conceptualized sexual behaviour as the outcome of natural, biological drives which form the basis for a variety of social experiences. Sexual normalcy and deviancy from the norm came to be defined in relation to the assumed biological naturalness of essential human reproductive instincts. As an instinctual and potentially overwhelming force, sex was at the same time seen as a possible source of social disorder. The Scottish 19th-century biologists Geddes and Thomson thus warned against the 'volcanic element in sex, quite underlying the rest of our nature and for that very reason shaking it from its foundations with tremors, if not catastrophe'. Consequently, it was argued, sexual instincts need to be kept in check by society through moral control, sex education, and legislation.

Pioneers of sexology such as the Germans Bloch, Krafft-Ebing, Hirschfeld, Westphal, Rohleder, Moll, and Friedländer, the Austrian Stekel, the French Féré and Thoinot, the Swiss Forel, the Hungarian Kaan, and the English Ellis set out to explore sexual 'abnormalcy' through zealous labelling and classification of deviations from the norm. They invented a wide range of new and increasingly exotic taxonomies of 'perversion', such as fetishism, sadomasochism, transvestism (also called eonism), hermaphrodism, frottage (rubbing against others), coprophilia (deriving sexual pleasure from faeces), necrophilia (sexual gratification from having sex with the dead), undinism (sexual arousal associated with water), algophilia (sexual gratification associated with inflicting or experiencing pain), and urolagnia (sexual pleasure from urinating), which they presented in 'the most nauseous detail', as a reviewer for the *British Medical Journal* described the case histories presented in Krafft-Ebing's influential medical handbook of sexual deviance *Psychopathia Sexualis* (1886). Sexology thus emerged in Europe as a new scientific discipline with international scope. It did not constitute, however, a homogeneous, unified field. Rather, it regrouped scientists with different institutional and political agendas, which led to controversies both within and in response to sexology. Public reactions were mixed. Some of the early works by Ellis and Bloch were prosecuted for obscenity, while Krafft-Ebing tactfully switched to Latin when describing specific sexual practices in *Psychopathia Sexualis* (rumours circulated at the time that sales of Latin dictionaries soared in Germany after the publication of his best-selling book).

Sexuality and gender differences

An important feature of this biological model was its biologization of gender difference. From the 18th century, the traditional idea of the 'one-sex body', which conceptualized women's bodies as similar but inferior versions of male bodies (with female genitals being thought of as internal, much smaller versions of male genitals), started to be replaced with the idea of a clear biological differentiation between men and women. Male and female bodies came to be seen as fundamentally, biologically different, not as part of the same hierarchical continuum. The gender hierarchy remained, however. It was variously based upon the amalgamation of femininity with motherhood, as in the 19th-century English evolutionist Herbert Spencer's claim that woman's inferior intellectual capacities were caused by the fact that she had stopped at an earlier stage of evolution in order to free energy to fulfil her role in the reproduction of the species; upon a claimed basic difference in 'cell metabolism', as the biologists Geddes and Thomson influentially argued; or upon hormonal differences between the sexes after the discovery of sex hormones around the turn of the 20th century. While claims about the biological inferiority of women were also used to legitimize the continued exclusion of women from the public sphere and politics in a context in which such exclusion became increasingly contested, the emergence of new ways of seeing the body transformed understandings of sex as well, as Laqueur has emphasized. Sex was no longer understood as an encounter between cold and hot, active and passive partners, but as an act between men and women who were now seen as biologically very different creatures.

The innate biological differences between men and women, which justified their assignment to different social roles, were thought also to lead to differences in sexual behaviour and needs. Whereas male sexuality was seen as naturally aggressive and forceful, women's sexuality was conceptualized as a response to male desire, driven by reproductive and maternal instincts. Although some sexologists, such as Havelock Ellis, emphasized the importance of female sexuality and of fulfilling sex as crucial for a happy life, the 19th-century English physician William Acton expressed prevalent public opinion when he stated:

> The majority of women are not much troubled by sexual feeling of any kind.

Sexologists routinely reproduced the double sexual morality of the time by picturing 'normal' women as passive and chaste, with a natural preference for monogamy, and by presenting male promiscuity as caused by 'the sexual demands of man's nature', as Krafft-Ebing put it. Consequently, 'excessive' sexual urges on the part of a woman were seen as abnormal. This resulted in a stark increase in the diagnosis of 'female hysteria' in the course of the 19th century, a nervous disorder that was thought to be caused by insufficient sexual satisfaction of excessively passionate women. Patients were sometimes treated by manual massage of their genitals by a doctor until 'hysterical paroxysm' (what contemporary terminology would describe as 'orgasm') occurred, while water massage devices were offered in spas across Europe and the United States and electrical vibrators became popular appliances with the spread of electricity to the private home. Alternatively, clitoridectomy could be proposed. Institutions across the US and the UK, such as the 'London Surgical Home for the Reception of Gentlewomen and Females of Respectability Suffering from Curable Surgical Diseases', set up in 1858, routinely offered clitoridectomy as a 'cure' for conditions ranging from hysteria to mania, idiocy, insanity, and urinary incontinence. Success stories circulated in England of operations performed on women who had sought divorce under the new 1857 Divorce Act, a behaviour that was interpreted as an obvious symptom of mental illness, and who after the operation conceded to return to their husbands. As the last example shows, genital mutilation could be used as an instrument for the disciplining of non-normative femininity.

Representations of female sexuality varied, however, with social class and race. Working-class girls and racial 'others' were often portrayed as more sexually available or even insatiable, as reflected in erotic literature such as John Cleland's *Fanny Hill* (1748) and the anonymous *My Secret Life* (1888), while prostitutes were commonly depicted as hypersexual beings with rotten, corrupted bodies. The lower categories were on the assumed hierarchical scale of civilization, the closer they were to 'primitives' – which is why, in general, women were assumed to be 'as a rule … much more the slaves of their instincts and habits than men', as the Swiss sexologist Auguste Forel put it. Working-class men and women, Africans, Asians, and Jews (the latter considered a separate 'race') were considered especially voluptuous and more likely to engage in 'uncivilized', 'degenerate' sexual practices.

Female sexuality remained an intense focus of problematization throughout the history of sexual science, though later sex research tended, on the contrary, to see lack of sexual desire or pleasure in women as pathological. An example of this can be found in the famous experimental research by the American sexologists Masters and Johnson on human sexual response, which included laboratory observation of the physiological responses of hundreds of men and women during masturbation and sexual intercourse from the late 1950s to 1990s. In line with many other sex researchers, Masters and Johnson observed that many women do not have orgasms from intercourse, coining the term female 'coital orgasmic inadequacy' in their best-selling *Human Sexual Inadequacy* (1970). Female sexuality was thus constructed as pathological in relation to male heterosexuality (although they also observed the capacity for women to have multiple orgasms).

Heterosexuality and 'perversion'

In addition to the biologization of gender differences, a further central feature of the biological model of sexuality was the assumption that 'natural' sexual behaviour included heterosexual acts and desires only. Heterosexuality was thus treated as the implicit norm, whereas homosexuality, in particular, came to be conceptualized as, somehow, an abnormal departure from the norm. However, when the American doctor James G. Kiernan adopted the term 'heterosexual' in its earliest-known occurrence in the English language, in a medical journal in 1892, he used it to describe the 'sexual perversion' of having sex for recreational rather than procreative reasons via 'abnormal methods of gratification', which referred to ensuring pleasure while avoiding reproduction. The association of heterosexuality with abnormal (i.e. non-procreative) craving for the opposite sex continued well into the 1920s, when an appetite for non-procreative different-sex sexuality started to be seen as the norm.

The biological model conceptualized people who engaged in deviant sexual practices as fundamentally different from others. This was an important conceptual innovation, which can be illustrated with the notion of the homosexual. Of course, same-sex practices have always occurred throughout history, and specific acts such as sodomy have been at times tolerated and at other times (most intensely in the 18th century) persecuted. However, any person – depending on their morality – was thought to be capable of such sinful practices. As Foucault famously pointed out, it was only much later, from the 19th century, that the idea started to emerge that people who engage in 'sodomy' are a separate type of person, with a specific identity and inclinations resulting from abnormal biological instincts which lead them to commit such acts: 'homosexuals'. As he put it,

> The sodomite had been a temporary aberration; the homosexual was now a species.

While some historians trace the beginnings of this change back to the late Middle Ages and point out that from the 17th and 18th centuries onwards a homosexual subculture, with specific meeting places, started to form in large European cities, it is certain that with the 19th-century conceptualization of the sodomite as a particular type of person, the modern homosexual was born. A Hungarian journalist born in Vienna, Karl-Maria Kertbeny, is generally credited with coining the term 'homosexual', first in a letter to Karl Heinrich Ulrichs, a German early advocate for the rights of sexual minorities, in 1868, then publicly in an anonymous pamphlet of 1869 campaigning against Prussian sodomy legislation. Kertbeny contrasted the homosexual initially with the 'monosexualist' (someone who masturbates), the 'heterogenit' (someone who has sex with animals), and the 'heterosexual' or 'normalsexual' (a man who has a sexual preference for women). On the latter category, Kertbeny held the view that the high sex drive of 'heterosexuals' or 'normalsexuals', which he claimed was stronger than that of homosexuals or bestialists, gave them an appetite for engaging in depraved excesses including incest, assaulting 'male but especially female minors', and 'behaving depravedly with corpses'. Given the later shift in meaning to denote the biological naturalness and moral superiority of heterosexuality, the invention of the category of the heterosexual in the context of Kertbeny's promotion of gay rights is 'one of sex history's grand ironies', as the historian Jonathan Ned Katz has pointed out.

The term 'homosexuality' was popularized in Germany by Krafft-Ebing and in the UK by Ellis. Charles Gilbert Chaddock, translator of Krafft-Ebing's *Psychopathia Sexualis*, is thus credited by the Oxford English Dictionary with having introduced the word 'homosexuality' into the English language in 1892, a year after a medical publication had introduced the same term into French. 'Lesbianism' first appeared in 1870, initially competing with the concepts of 'tribadism' or 'sapphism'. The term 'homosexual' also had early competitors. The German pioneering campaigner for sexual rights Karl Heinrich Ulrichs, for example, founded in 1862 the cult of 'Uranism', a term borrowed from Plato's *Symposium* in which 'Uranian' or 'heavenly' love of men for boys, attributed to the god Uranus, is praised. Against the backdrop of the romanticist rediscovery of ancient Greece in Germany and Victorian England, other Uranian societies promoting male love and friendship sprang up in both countries, including in Oxford and Cambridge. Other terminological contenders were 'homosexualist'; 'paederast' (though referring to sex with boys, it came to be used also to refer to sex between men); 'contrary sexual feeling'; 'inverted sexual proclivity'; 'sexual inversion'; 'intermediate sex'; 'third sex'; and 'urnings' (again, from 'Uranian love').

The concept of 'sexual inversion' was particularly popular in the 19th century. It expressed the widespread belief of the time that people with same-sex desires suffered from some kind of gender disorder and were really women in men's bodies, or vice versa (though the concept also covered a wider range of deviant gender behaviours such as men dressing up in women's clothes), or even a third sex. Same-sex desire was widely interpreted through the lens of gender, but disagreements raged over what the exact link between sexual identity and gender was. Whereas those defending the sexual inversion model argued that male homosexuals were 'feminized', others held up the Greek paederastic model to argue that they were, on the contrary, especially masculine. The first movement for the rights of sexual minorities in the world emerged in Germany around the end of the 19th century, following the criminalization of homosexuality at a national scale that had resulted from German unification. By 1902, divisions within the movement emerged over precisely this question, with Magnus Hirschfeld defending the third-sex model, whereas Benedict Friedländer argued that homosexuality was 'the highest, most perfect evolutionary stage of gender differentiation', and that the 'inverted type' of male homosexual represented hypervirility, and possessed superior capacities for leadership and heroism than did heterosexual men.

In both competing models, homosexual men and women were considered to be biologically separate types of individuals from heterosexuals, with specific personality traits, clothes, and bodies, and it was claimed that they were particularly prevalent in large urban centres (which, in the context of the social disruptions resulting from accelerating urbanization processes, were held to be particularly fertile breeding grounds for perversion, compared to the simple, 'natural' life in the countryside).

The biological model of sexuality saw homosexuals not as sinners or criminals, but as abnormal individuals who were in need of a cure. Although some sexologists, including Ellis, saw homosexuality as inborn but not a disease, much of sexual science has been preoccupied with problematizing and investigating these 'marginal' sexualities, and with thinking about how to 'correct' the perceived pathologies through therapy, and chemical and surgical interventions, including castration. Homosexuality was officially classified as a mental illness in the American Psychiatric Association's Diagnostic and Statistical Manual until 1973, and by the World Health Organization until 1992. Similar psychiatric labels were abolished in the UK in 1994, in the Russian Federation in 1999, and by the Chinese Society of Psychiatry in 2001, after gay rights groups as well as dissenting psychiatrists argued that homophobia rather than homosexuality was the problem.

The use of psychiatry and sexology to correct and cure deviant sexuality has been widely documented. For example, psychoanalysts such as the American Sandor Rado argued from the 1940s that deviancy from heterosexuality could be 'unlearned'. By the 1950s and 1960s, aversion therapy was increasingly used to 'cure' sexual deviants such as cross-dressers, fetishists, transsexuals, homosexuals, and lesbians in countries including the Soviet Union, the UK, the US, Canada, and South Africa. Gay men were more frequently targeted than lesbians since therapeutic treatment would often be part of criminal sentences, which only rarely involved lesbian relationships. The US sexologists Masters and Johnson ran a programme from 1968 to 1977 to convert homosexuals to heterosexuality, with a claimed success rate of 71.6% over six years of treatment. Aversion therapy involved projecting images of 'inappropriate sexual objects', including current lovers, to the 'patient', who was then injected with chemicals such as apomorphine to cause nausea and vomiting, or subjected to electric shock treatments which would commonly be administered two or more times daily over a period of several weeks.

Although sexologists themselves often promoted tolerance for those who fell outside of the 'normalcy' of heterosexual relationships, their ideas were also used to organize and intensify the emerging disciplining of sexuality. As the sociologist Jeffrey Weeks puts it:

[T]he paradox was that the early sexologists, who by and large were also conscious sex reformers, were simultaneously powerful agents in the organisation, and potential control, of the sexual behaviours they sought to describe.

Indeed, many of the pioneers of sexual science were active social reformers who saw sexual reform and the transformation of the social order as connected. This was true, for example, of figures such as Auguste Forel, Edward Carpenter, Havelock Ellis, Richard von Krafft-Ebing, Magnus Hirschfeld, and Iwan Bloch who were actively involved in political campaigns that ranged from the rights of sexual minorities to pacifism and votes for women. Against the backdrop of such wider social struggles, they participated in contemporary and highly politicized public debates on sex reform, sex education, and discriminatory legislation. Many early sexologists saw homosexuals in particular as 'harmless', especially since, as Auguste Forel remarked, 'they would not reproduce anyway', and authors such as Krafft-Ebing and Hirschfeld spoke out publicly against anti-sodomy legislation.

Sexual revolution

The politicization of sexuality was intensified in the 1960s, when Freudian Marxists such as Herbert Marcuse, Erich Fromm, and Wilhelm Reich argued that sex is a natural, positive force that is repressed by bourgeois capitalist society, and called for sexual 'liberation' which would transform the social order. Wilhelm Reich was an Austrian psychoanalyst who in the 1920s and 1930s was a member, first, of the Austrian social-democrat party, then of the German communist party, before becoming a fervent critic of the 'red fascism' of communism in the 1940s and 1950s, by which time he had emigrated to the US. Reich's early and most influential work tried to reconcile psychoanalysis with Marxism. He built upon Freud's emphasis on the importance of libido (sexual energy) but took issue with Freud's theory, stated most explicitly in *Civilisation and Its Discontents* (1915), that the subject achieves 'normal' adult identity by redirecting the libido into other areas of life. Whereas, for Freud, culture thus advances as a result of the suppression of nature, for Reich culture and nature, while pitted in opposition in modern society, should instead be reconciled in a state of mutual harmony. Reich proposed a 'correction of Freud's theory of the unconscious' by turning Freud's ideas on sexuality on their head and suggesting, in his own theories of 'vegetotherapy' and, later, 'sex-economy', that it was the cultural repression of natural, sexual energy that was the origin of all neurosis. As he put it in 1948:

> My contention is that every individual who has managed to preserve a bit of naturalness knows that there is only one thing wrong with neurotic patients: the lack of full and repeated sexual satisfaction.

Whereas Reich saw full 'orgastic potency', which he identified with 'genital gratification', as a biological capacity, he argued that this natural ability for genital pleasure had been destroyed by society. 'A sex-economist', he declared, '... knows that man is the only biological species which has destroyed its own natural sex function, and that is what ails him.' This destruction of orgastic potency was all the more preoccupying as sexuality 'is the life energy *per se*', as he put it, and as it was so widespread. Indeed, Reich argued that the majority of individuals suffer from sexual repression in modern society. As he wrote:

> Not a single neurotic individual possesses orgastic potency; the corollary of this fact is the fact that the vast majority of humans suffer from a character-neurosis.

Reich's most influential writings thus developed analyses of the ways in which society turned individuals into neurotics, putting the responsibility for this 'mass neurosis' at first on capitalism, later on authoritarian society, and in his final work on any social institutions which repressed the biological life energy. The institution of the 'authoritarian compulsive family' as incarnated in the nuclear family model came in for particular criticism, since it reproduced in Reich's eyes the authoritarian structures of the state at the micro-level, and propped up the social, economic, and sexual oppression of women by patriarchy. Denouncing the compulsive monogamy that created so much spousal unhappiness, and the economic dependency of women and children within the family, Reich also saw the family as a central agent in the social repression of natural childhood and adolescent sexual exploration. Reich called for a 'sexual revolution' which would liberate sexuality from its suppression by society – something that would not be possible, he believed, without overthrowing the social and political order as well. As he wrote in the preface to the second edition of his 1930 work *The Sexual Revolution*:

[A]uthoritarian social order and social sexual suppression go hand in hand, and revolutionary 'morality' and gratification of the sexual needs go together.

Reich's earlier, mostly sexological and psychological, notion of sex-economy was in his later decades rephrased as the science of 'orgonomy', the study of 'life energy'. Having moved to the US in 1939, Reich set up a research centre called 'Orgonon' in rural Maine. Having long argued that 'the genital sexual function' is the central source of life energy, he claimed to have identified, by observation, the origin of all life: cosmic orgone energy. Moving from a sociological and anthropological approach towards a natural science one to the study of life energy, Reich would stretch the patience of even his most fervent followers to its limits by his claims that the 'particles of life energy', which he called the 'bion', as well as life-destroying particles, which he called 'Deadly Orgone' or 'DOR', could be observed experimentally; by his 'discovery' of the chemical formula of the unconscious; and by his invention of cloud-busting machines which he claimed could draw upon orgone energy to produce rain. His most controversial invention was that of energy accumulators called 'orgone boxes', which he claimed could channel cosmic orgone energy to individuals sitting in these boxes. Orgone energy could, he claimed, deblock people's 'bio-energy', the stagnation of which in modern society he saw as the origin of 'orgasm anxiety' as well as contributing to a number of ailments including cancer.

The orgone accumulators got Reich into trouble with the Federal Food and Drug Administration, however. An investigation into the suspected fraudulence of the claims of their health benefits led to a formal complaint on behalf of the FDA and a legal injunction against any reference to 'orgone energy'. Following a technical violation of the injunction, Reich was sentenced in 1956 to a two-year prison term, the banning of references to orgone energy and accumulators in his books, and the burning of material related to the accumulators. He was to die in a federal penitentiary in Pennsylvania a year later. Presently, by way of contrast, orgone accumulators are freely on sale on the Internet.

The call for sexual liberation from capitalist and patriarchal repression by the Freudian Left was to have a deep influence on the leftist and feminist movements that emerged in the 1960s and 1970s, as well as on various new types of sex therapy which promoted the release of sexual energy. It reproduced a biological understanding of sexuality as a natural force, repressed by bourgeois society.

The biological model remained dominant up until the 1980s and is still an important theoretical influence on sex research today, especially given the current revival of evolutionary models of sexuality and genetic perspectives. For example, books such as Randy Thornhill and Craig Palmer's *A Natural History of Rape: Biological Bases of Sexual Coercion* (2000) and Michael Ghiglieri's *The Dark Side of Man* (1999) conceptualize male sexual violence, in particular rape, as the result of evolutionary male instincts to spread their genes, while Helen Fisher's *Anatomy of Love: A Natural History of Mating, Marriage and Why We*

Stray (1992) points at evolutionary and biological explanations of gender differences. However, the biological model of sexuality has come under attack from various quarters, including from within sexology itself.

Challenges to the biological model of sex

Although most early sexologists primarily explored the peripheral sexualities, others, in particular Havelock Ellis, focused on 'normal' sexual behaviour itself. The study of normative sexuality led to the partial problematization of biological naturalness. Sex was still understood in terms of biological essence, but some 19th-century sexologists, such as Geddes and Thomson, could not help noticing that 'natural' sexual instincts were, in fact, quite diverse. Even among the first generation of sexologists, the naturalizing account of sexual orthodoxy thus simultaneously led to a partial problematization of sexual normalcy. The suggestion by Ellis that normality itself reflected social definitions rather than natural instincts, and that there might be a continuum rather than a sharp break between normal and abnormal sexual practices, opened up the path for social understandings of sexuality.

Later sex research involved large-scale surveys and statistical analysis of sexual attitudes and behaviours in numerous countries. The best-known examples of these are the 1950s studies of the sexual behaviour of 12,000 Americans by Kinsey, and the successive Hite reports which surveyed the sexual experiences of 15,000 men and women in the US from the 1970s onwards. Again, an important consequence of these naturalistic, quantitative surveys of sexual attitudes and behaviour was to show that the frontiers between 'normal' and 'deviant' sexuality are not as clear-cut as had previously been thought. Kinsey's studies in particular created public scandal in the early 1950s, when they revealed that 37% of the male sample had engaged in sex to orgasm with another man, most of whom considered themselves as heterosexuals – a finding that is fairly routine in contemporary surveys of sexual behaviour. This meant that same-sex activity could no longer be labelled as the deviant behaviour of a small, diseased minority of people. It is an important paradox in the history of sexology that while the biological model conceptualized sexuality in terms of natural instincts, normal and abnormal sexuality, and biological gender differences, the same type of research has also led to the problematization of the very categories that it was based upon. The biological understanding of sexuality was thus challenged from within the sexological discourse that had formulated it in the first place.

The biological model was also challenged by the very subjects that it endeavoured to describe. Within the 'peripheral' sexualities that sexual science created, sexual meanings have been experimented on and contested. As Jeffrey Weeks points out:

> [T]he speaking perverts, first given a carefully shaded public platform in the volumes of early sexologists, have become highly vocal on their behalf. ... They speak for themselves in street politics and lobbying, through pamphlets, journals and books, via the semiotics of highly sexualised settings, with their elaborate codes of keys, colours and clothes, in the popular media, and in the more mundane details of domestic life.

Taxonomic labels such as 'homosexual' or 'lesbian' have been re-appropriated in politically creative ways by the categories to which they were initially applied, as we shall see later (see p. 102).

A third major challenge to the biological model came from Freud. He developed a theory of unconscious drive/libido that saw sexual desire not as something that could be controlled and overcome, but as ever-present in men as well as women. Within this framework, he portrayed female hysteria as a symptom of the unhealthy repression of female sexual instincts. His influential *Three Essays on the Theory of Sexuality* (1905) conceptualized sexuality not as a pre-given, ready-made natural instinct from which subjects can then deviate, but rather as a drive that is constructed in the process of childhood psychological development. Freud argued that the channelling of the child's diffuse sexuality into socially acceptable forms is central to its development into adulthood. As the Freudian feminist Juliet Mitchell puts it:

> [I]n childhood all is diverse or perverse; unification and 'normality' are the effort we must make on our entry into human society.

While placing central importance upon sexuality by seeing human agency as driven by unconscious desire, Freud's analyses of individual cases of hysteria and neurosis moved away from biological accounts, linking civilization and sexual repression.

The final and possibly most decisive challenge to the biological model of sexuality has resulted from the emergence of anti-essentialist perspectives across a range of disciplines in the social sciences and the humanities from the 1970s onwards. These new theoretical models reject the idea of sexuality as natural or biological, emphasizing instead the social nature of sexual experience. Following Foucault's controversial but highly influential account, in his canonical *History of Sexuality: An Introduction*, of sexuality as a 'historical apparatus' whose origins can be retraced to the 18th century, authors such as David Halperin in classics, Stephen Heath in literary criticism, and Jeffrey Weeks, Ken Plummer, and numerous others in sociology have argued prominently for the need to understand sexuality as a historically and culturally situated domain of experience that is shaped by social relations of power. Following this social model of sexuality, sexual identities are not merely the expression of natural instincts, but are social as well as political constructs.

Against this backdrop, the claim that heterosexuality, homosexuality, lesbianism, and even sexuality itself were invented in the 19th century does not mean merely that the terms were invented in that period (although they were). More fundamentally, it means that the ways in which individuals experience and make sense of their sexualities and identities in modernity are heavily shaped by the core elements associated with the conceptual apparatus of sexuality, in particular the idea of 'natural' sexual instinct, the assumed biological basis for gender differences, and the notion of sexual identity.

As we have seen, cultural understandings of sex have, in the West, been shaped by three models: the moral/religious model, the biological model, and the social model of sexuality. Although these three models have, historically, emerged successively, it is important to emphasize that they are still co-present today. Moral, biological, and social understandings of sexuality continue to have a great influence on the ways in which sexual meanings are organized in society, politics, and in our everyday lives. They have important implications for the ways in which we conceptualize our sexual behaviours and identities, as well as the possibilities for personal and political transformation.

Chapter 3
Virgins or whores? Feminist critiques of sexuality

Feminists who still sleep with the man are delivering their most
vital energies to the oppressor.

Jill Johnson, *Lesbian Nation* (1973)

The double moral standard

Female sexuality has been subjected to particular scientific and
moral scrutiny throughout modernity. It has also constituted a
central concern in feminist struggles. While the first women's
movement that emerged in the last decades of the 19th century
prioritized the fight for civic and political equality for women,
sexuality constituted nevertheless an important area for the
critique of existing gender relations. Drawing on biological
justifications of the double moral standard which saw men
as naturally promiscuous and women as passive and chaste,
feminists built upon such views of gender to argue that women's
morals were consequently by nature superior to those of men.
Occupying the moral high ground, they developed a critique of
male sexuality which pointed at the natural lustful drives of men
and male sexual freedom as the origin of the sexual oppression
of women. Reflecting wider social concerns of the time about the
expansion of prostitution in the 19th century across Europe and
the US, and the attendant increase in venereal disease, political

activism centred especially on these areas. The 'real' reason why men did not wish to give women the vote, some feminists argued, was to protect male sexual exploitation of women.

Female activists from mostly upper-middle-class backgrounds played important roles in the numerous social movements promoting greater moral purity and 'social hygiene' that emerged both from the political Left and from conservative and religious organizations across the Western world. Campaigns against prostitution called for an end to the 'white slavery' which forced innocent, impoverished young working-class girls into sexual exploitation by unscrupulous middle-class men. Instead, they promoted 'rescue work' for 'fallen women'. The moralist view was that prostitution was a vice; it was also considered a major public health problem. Prostitutes were seen as the main vehicles of the contamination of men with venereal diseases such as gonorrhoea and syphilis, echoing traditional associations in Western culture between the female body and disease. As Shakespeare's mad King Lear put it:

Down from the waist they are all Centaurs,
Though women all above;
But to the girdle do the Gods inherit,
Beneath is all the fiend's; there's hell, there's darkness,
There is the sulphurous pit – burning, scalding,
Stench, consumption; fie, fie, fie! Pah, pah!

Venereal disease itself came to be culturally represented as female in the modern age, as 'Dame Syphilis' as the French called it. Syphilis had appeared in Europe from the late 15th century, possibly spread by sailors returning from the Americas, and led to an epidemic across the continent. Collective anxieties about syphilis portrayed it as coming from the 'outside', in particular from foreigners, reflecting wider cultural meanings around sexual disease which tended to see the healthy, male bodies of the nation as polluted by diseased female and foreign bodies. As the medical author Llewellyn-Jones has pointed out:

> As the people of each country became infected, each tried to put the blame for the new and terrifying disease on its neighbour. The Italians called it the Spanish disease. The French, who were first infected in 1495, called it the Italian or Neapolitan disease... It reached England in 1497, where it was called the French disease... It reached China in 1505 and Japan a year later where it was called 'manka bassam' or the Portuguese disease.

Sexually transmitted disease carried associations of foreign invasion and treason. During the First and Second World Wars, prostitutes were thus routinely portrayed as 'helping the enemy' by contaminating patriotic soldiers. A widely diffused British Second World War poster carried a picture of a skull-faced prostitute linking arms with Hitler and Hirohito, accompanied by the caption 'VD worst of the three'. Thousands of suspected prostitutes were jailed in internment camps in the US during the First World War, and Magnus Hirschfeld's *The Sexual History of the World War* (1941) reports that the German army issued edicts in several occupied territories in 1915 punishing women who had sex with soldiers while knowingly infected with VD with sentences of up to a year in prison.

Driven by fears that venereal disease would make male bodies too weak for military purposes, many national states started to regulate prostitution in the 19th century in order to limit the spread of sexual infections. No efforts were made to prevent customers from contaminating prostitutes, but the latter were targeted with compulsory medical inspection, and, if contamination was diagnosed, incarceration and forced hospital treatment ensued. Folk beliefs circulated in 19th-century Europe that intercourse with a child virgin could cure venereal disease. More generally, child prostitution was widespread across Europe and elsewhere, though it was common for virginity to be faked so that a girl could be sold at a higher price several times over. An international scandal was caused by the publication of a series of highly graphic accounts of the entrapment and sale of young girls in London brothels by the journalist W. T. Stead in the *Pall Mall Gazette* in July 1885. The series, published under the name 'The Maiden Tribute of Modern Babylon', uncovered a sexual underworld where upper-class gentlemen could revel in the 'cries of tortured victims of lust and brutality'. It led, in the UK, to the 1885 Criminal Law Amendment Act which criminalized procurement and raised the age of sexual consent for girls from 13 to 16.

In alliance with Christian organizations, 19th-century feminist anti-prostitution campaigners called upon national states not to regulate but to ban prostitution altogether. State regulation meant, they argued, that the state 'acted like a pimp' by maintaining the institution of prostitution. In 1875, a major international movement was founded in the shape of the British and Continental Federation for the Abolition of Government Regulation of Vice, which called for the abolition of prostitution. High on its political agenda was the fight against the international traffic in women for the purposes of prostitution, reflecting wider social panics of the time concerning the effects on society of increasing immigration patterns. In 1904, the first 'International Agreement for the Suppression of the White Slave Traffic' was agreed upon, giving rise to a gradual process of legal prohibition of brothels across most Western countries.

First-wave feminist campaigns mobilized both the moral and the biological model of sexuality to argue for the need to protect women from the dire consequences of male lust. They placed women in the role of guardians of public and private morality, thereby reproducing the prevalent social models of femininity of the time, which based female respectability on virginal purity or married chastity, while the immoral, 'depraved' behaviour of sexually promiscuous women defined them as 'whores' either metaphorically or literally.

Free love

Not all feminists shared this binary view of female sexuality, however. Numerous prominent feminist thinkers participated in 19th-century radical sex reform movements which argued for greater sexual freedoms for men as well as women. Libertarian, anarchist, and communist thinkers attacked obscenity and anti-homosexuality laws, calling for access to birth control information, abortion, and 'free love' between equal partners within a freely chosen bond. Echoing earlier attacks on the institution of marriage by feminist pioneers such as Mary Wollstonecraft, they rejected the marriage contract as founded upon the economic and physical appropriation of women by men, though most free love thinkers encouraged monogamous relationships. Free love was promoted by freethinkers, anarchists, and socialist feminists such as the Americans Emma Goldman and Lillian Harman, or Ito Noe in Japan, who was murdered with her male lover by Japanese military police in 1923. The German *Verband Fortschrittlicher Frauenvereine* (League of Progressive Women's Associations) proposed a boycott of marriage and celebrated sexual pleasure for women as well as men, while the English Legitimation League, originally created in 1893 for the defence of the rights of children born out of wedlock, called for the merging together of 'two of the noblest principles of human relations – freedom and love'. Alexandra Kollontai, the most prominent female communist revolutionary in the early decades of the Soviet state and founder of the *Zhenotdel* (Women's section of the Central Committee of the Bolshevik Party) in 1919, argued that the family, like the state, was a capitalist institution which would wither away with the future development of the socialist 'heaven on earth'. 'The family', she wrote in 1920, 'is ceasing to be necessary either to its members or to the nation as a whole.' As she put it in her 1920 text *Communism and the Family*:

> Instead of the conjugal slavery of the past, communist society offers women and men a free union which is strong in the comradeship which inspired it.

Since female sexual exploitation was linked to the economic dependency of women on men of the capitalist system, prostitution, she believed, would also 'automatically disappear' in the radiant communist future. The sex drive, which she saw 'not as something shameful and sinful but as something which is as natural as the other needs of a healthy organism, such as hunger and thirst', should not be restrained as long as sexual excess, which threatened workers' capacity for productivity, was avoided, as she wrote in her 1921 text *Theses on Communist Morality in the Sphere of Marital Relations*.

Kollontai's views were rapidly sidelined by Lenin, while free love thinkers in capitalist societies generally encountered hostility from mainstream suffragist organizations which feared that sexual libertarianism would undermine the social respectability of wider campaigns for women's rights (much as socialist organizations generally feared that support for 'free love' would alienate their working-class members). Sexual radicals and mainstream feminists agreed, however, on women's right to refuse 'unreasonable' male sexual demands and excessive numbers of pregnancies, and to ownership over their own bodies, promoting the concept of 'voluntary motherhood'. Whereas some saw the solution in greater access to sex education and contraceptive information and methods, others called upon men to exercise greater self-control and chastity, leading the Victorian physician William Acton to complain in 1871:

> During the last few years, and since the rights of women have been so much insisted upon ... numerous husbands have complained to me of the hardships under which they suffer by being married to women who regard themselves as martyrs when called upon to

fullfill the duties of wives. This spirit of insubordination has become intolerable.

Free love feminists saw the liberation of sexuality as crucial for a wider transformation in the social position of women, in a context in which there was no legal abortion, methods of birth control were largely unreliable, mortality rates of women in childbirth or from backstreet abortions were high, and women were profoundly dependent upon men.

Sexual liberation

The women's movements that emerged in the 1960s and 1970s, generally referred to as 'second-wave feminism', put the politicization of sexuality at the heart of their agenda, but did so in an entirely different social context. Second-wave women's movements emerged in societies whose traditional gender relations had been fundamentally transformed by the massive post-war entry of women into the workforce. Against the backdrop of greater economic independence that resulted both from women's entry into paid work and from the emerging state provision of welfare which offered alternative support mechanisms, wider (and partly linked) detraditionalization processes occurred which transformed the institutions of marriage, the family, and gender. Overall, women's control over their own life options increased significantly, especially for middle-class women; though rising divorce rates also produced a feminization of poverty, primarily among single mothers in those countries where welfare state support was weakest.

Meanwhile, a further major set of social changes took place in the area of reproductive control. The prominent American birth control campaigner (and eugenicist) Margaret Sanger, founder of the American Birth Control League in 1921, had long called for the development of a pharmaceutical birth control product, meeting up with scientists in 1950 to explore possibilities. Sanger joined forces with the philanthropist Katherine McCormick, who funded the majority of the scientific research and development of the Pill, and from 1960 the modern contraceptive pill, invented by Karl Djerassi, became available to the wider public in the Western world. With the availability of reliable birth control for the first time in human history, and the subsequent elaboration of new reproductive technologies such as IVF (in vitro fertilization) which mean that conception cannot just be prevented but also artificially produced, Freud's famous claim that 'anatomy is destiny' is no longer true. And yet, many feminists initially received the Pill with hostile suspicion. They considered it as another example of male medical control over female bodies, especially given the negative side effects of the initially highly dosed new product.

The uncoupling of intercourse and reproduction involved a radical transformation of the conditions of female sexuality with, in turn, profound consequences for male sexuality. How far access to contraception encouraged the sexual revolution of the 1960s and 1970s has been hotly contested, but it was certainly an important precondition. The rise of sexual permissiveness and the emergence of new meanings around love, sex, and relationships, which spread from the pioneering countries of the Netherlands, Sweden, and Denmark across the Western world, transformed the landscape of sexuality. The countercultural social movements that emerged in the 1960s, most prominently the American Civil Rights and anti-war movements with their slogan 'make love not war', as well as the anti-authoritarian student movements in countries such as France, Germany, the Netherlands, and the UK, were heavily influenced by sexual liberation theorists such as Fromm, Reich, and Marcuse. They promoted the liberation of 'natural' sexual desire from bourgeois repression as part of a wider project of political subversion of capitalist, authoritarian society.

Symbolized by the 'summer of love' of 1967, the increase in sexual permissiveness has conventionally been interpreted by sociologists such as Anthony Giddens to be 'gender-neutral', and to have led to greater female sexual autonomy. Many feminists initially embraced the sexual revolution with great enthusiasm, seeing sexual liberation as crucial for women's liberation generally. From the end of the 1960s, consciousness-raising groups sprang up in many countries which encouraged women to explore their bodies and capacities for sexual pleasure, such as the 'bodysex workshops' that the sex educator Betty Dodson organized from 1973 in the US. Having presented female masturbation as a means of reversing the repression of female sexuality in her book *Liberating Masturbation*, Dodson's workshops guided a circle of naked participants in collective 'orgasm rituals' with the help of vibrators. Dodson further celebrated 'swinging' and campaigned against monogamous possessiveness, jealousy, and sexual guilt – ideas that were promoted with considerable enthusiasm by many other sexual revolutionaries at the time. *More Joy of Sex*, for example, the follow-up of the international best-selling sex manual *The Joy of Sex* (1972) written for a mainstream public by the sexologist Alex Comfort, presented a positive picture of swinging among members of a community, though it warned against choosing to do it with close friends or with strangers (while later editions warned against swinging altogether, on the grounds of HIV/Aids risk).

The sexual revolution was nothing like the 'fulfilling love and sex between equal partners' which the free love feminists had imagined, however. The cultural transformations involved in the sexual revolution were primarily led by men, and largely reproduced the unequal relations of power between men and women while celebrating a normative promiscuity which, feminist critics suggested, benefited men more than women. Works such as Sheila Jeffreys's *Anticlimax: A Feminist Perspective on the Sexual Revolution*, published in 1990, argued that, in retrospect, the revolution was less an increase in sexual freedom for women than the fulfilment of male fantasies about female availability. The rhetoric of sexual liberation legitimized male control of women's sexuality and made it impossible to 'say no' to sexual advances, they claimed. As feminist author Beatrix Campbell put it in 1980:

> ... the permissive era had some pay-off for women in so far as it opened up political-sexual-space. It permitted sex for women too. What it did not do was defend women against the differential effects of permissiveness on men and women ... It was about the affirmation of young men's sexuality and promiscuity; (...) The very affirmation of sexuality was a celebration of *masculine* sexuality.

Nor was the sexual revolution quite what Marxist liberation theorists had pictured. Far from the subversion of capitalism by the free reign of the pleasure principle which Marcuse and Reich had hoped for, the lifting of obscenity and other morality laws that resulted from the relaxation of moral controls over sexuality opened the floodgates to the commodification of sex at a previously unprecedented scale. The national and international sex industry dramatically expanded, and it became a major player in the capitalist global economy. Whereas *The Joy of Sex* had predicted that sexual freedom would render prostitution unnecessary, since women would now be willing to meet all male sexual needs for free, commercial sex in reality greatly increased – as did pornography. Both prostitution and pornography consequently rapidly returned to the agenda of the women's movement.

The politics of orgasm

More generally, sexuality became one of the central issues of second-wave feminism. The sexual oppression of women came to be seen as a central – by some theorists, as *the* most central – area of male power over women. The new women's movement thus adopted the slogan 'the personal is political', expressing the idea that many of women's 'personal' life experiences are in fact rooted in the subordinated position that women as a group have within the gendered power structure. Consciousness-raising groups that aimed to increase awareness of the structural basis of individual women's experiences were consequently seen as an important basis for collective political action. Within the context of this politicization of the 'private', sexuality was intensely discussed and problematized. It was central to an important part of feminist theory and activism since the 1970s, including issues such as the right to sexual pleasure, the right to say 'no', political lesbianism, and debates around contraception, abortion, rape, sexual abuse, pornography, prostitution, and sexual harassment; most of the issues that mainstream politics had conventionally defined as part of the 'private' sphere of the family and the individual citizen. Feminist activism undertook to introduce the politics of sex into the political arena – and generally succeeded.

The feminist problematization of sexuality did not, however, constitute a unified whole. Since Kate Millett's *Sexual Politics* (1970), multiple and diverging voices have participated and contributed to the debates on sexuality. Disagreements on the role of sexuality in relations of power between men and women led to both political and theoretical differences in analysis. Influential socialist feminists such as Zillah Eisenstein, Michèle Barrett, and Juliet Mitchell, or the French 1970s '*Psych et Po*' (psychoanalysis and politics) group, turned towards Marxism, Freudianism, or a mix of the two to explore sexual repression and its links to capitalism. Others rejected psychoanalysis altogether for its perceived fundamental misogyny, while the Marxist assumption that the exploitation of women would come to an end with the withering away of the state was dismissed on the grounds that 'we cannot wait that long', as Germaine Greer put it in the *Female Eunuch* (1971). Alternative perspectives emerged over the next decades, including post-structuralist, postmodern, and postcolonial analyses of gender and sexuality, which currently compete with psychoanalytical and materialist/post-Marxist theory.

One of the most prominent theoretical battlegrounds over competing theories of female sexuality emerged within sexology. For a long time, sex research had considered female sexuality as a simple response to male instincts, as we have seen in Chapter 2. By investigating female sexuality as an autonomous research object, the US sexologist Kinsey opened up new ways of studying and of interpreting both male and female sexuality. This path was further pursued by sexologists like Masters and Johnson, Fisher, Kaplan, Sherfey, and Hite, as well as Friday's best-selling series of studies on male and female sexual fantasies. The study of female sexuality was particularly marked by controversies around female orgasm and its link to female anatomy. The emerging women's movement enthusiastically welcomed the research of sexologists Masters and Johnson whose laboratory observation of over 10,000 male and female orgasms in the 1960s had revealed women's virtually unlimited orgasmic capacities. In their 1970 work *The Pleasure Bond*, Masters and Johnson – who had already described themselves as 'not remotely' feminists a few years earlier – had equated women's liberation with sexual liberation and argued against the double moral standard which, they argued, taught women more than men to repress their sexual desires. Their rehabilitation of the important role of the clitoris for female sexual pleasure contrasted to much previous sexual science, which had traditionally emphasized the superiority and naturalness (or, as some strands of psychoanalysis argued, the greater maturity) of vaginal orgasm. Marie Bonaparte, for example, the most prominent promoter of Freud's ideas in France, thus proposed in the 1950s a surgical intervention which would locate the clitoris closer to the vagina as a cure for frigidity, in order to make 'defective' female anatomy fit better with Freudian assumptions about 'mature' sexuality. The sexologist Frank Caprio expressed widely held views when he stated in his 1963 book *The Sexually Adequate Woman*:

> ...whenever a woman is incapable of achieving an orgasm via coitus, provided the husband is an adequate partner, and prefers clitoral

stimulation to any other form of sexual activity, she can be regarded as suffering from frigidity and requires psychiatric assistance.

Anne Koedt's influential essay 'The Myth of the Vaginal Orgasm' opened feminist attacks on such views in 1970, arguing that:

> Women have thus been defined sexually in terms of what pleases men; our own biology has not been properly analysed. Instead, we are fed the myth of the liberated woman and her vaginal orgasm – an orgasm which in fact does not exist.

Women who claimed to have vaginal orgasms were either faking or 'confused', Koedt controversially argued. The normative emphasis on vaginal orgasm in psychoanalysis and sexual science thus came to stand for male oppression of female sexuality for feminists, and became an important issue in the politicization of sex. The gender politics of orgasm was particularly central to the work of feminist sexologist Shere Hite, whose series of studies on male and female sexuality became international bestsellers, especially *The Hite Report on Female Sexuality* (1976) and *The Hite Report on Male Sexuality* (1981). As Hite put it in the report on female sexuality:

> Lack of sexual satisfaction is another sign of the oppression of women.

The Hite reports were based on wide-scale sexual surveys among women and men. Among the surveys' most hotly debated findings, the report on women observed that 'only approximately 30 percent of the women in this study could orgasm regularly from intercourse'; a result that in itself was not new. Sexual science had long been preoccupied with the lack of enthusiasm that many women seemed to have for intercourse, and earlier surveys by Kinsey, Masters and Johnson, and others had already found that the majority of women do not orgasm from intercourse alone. Hite used her result, however, to challenge the dominant sexological understanding of sexuality which reduced sexuality to heterosexual intercourse, and had consequently arrived at the conclusion that the great majority of women are 'frigid'.

Masters and Johnson were among the main targets of Hite's criticism. Despite their revaluation of clitoral orgasm, Masters and Johnson portrayed 'normal' sexuality as involving orgasm from intercourse and argued that the clitoris was automatically stimulated during intercourse by the 'mechanical traction' caused by 'active penile thrusting' – leading the feminist Alix Shulman to comment: 'much, I suppose, as a penis is automatically "stimulated" by a man's underwear whenever he takes a step'. For those men and women who did not respond to this 'natural' model, Masters and Johnson pioneered new types of sex therapy that aimed to teach subjects to overcome their 'dysfunction' by 'putting sex back in its natural context', that is, by training them to reach orgasm from intercourse. According to Masters' own estimate, within five years of the publication of *Human Sexual Inadequacy*, between 3,500 and 5,000 clinics offering treatment for sex problems were established in the US. Masters and Johnson revolutionized the sex therapy methods used in such clinics by providing 'incredibly vulnerable unmarried' men, as they described them, with female surrogate partners for treatment of male sexual 'inadequacy'. They did not, however, provide male surrogates to sexually inadequate unmarried women, on the grounds that this would be in conflict with the 'sexual value systems' of the time, and they later abandoned the use of surrogates altogether after being sued by an irate husband whose wife had volunteered to work as a surrogate.

Hite pointed out that most women seem more than capable of experiencing orgasm, only not via intercourse. Indeed, the majority of women in her survey seemed perfectly capable of procuring pleasure to their body by stimulating themselves, she remarked. 'Of the 82 percent of women who say they masturbated', Hite wrote, '95 percent could orgasm easily and regularly, whenever they wanted.' Women's problem was consequently not what Masters and Johnson termed female 'coital orgasmic inadequacy', but rather the way in which society defined sexual norms, in Hite's view:

> The fact that women can orgasm easily and pleasurably whenever they want (many women several times in a row) shows beyond a doubt that women *know* how to enjoy their bodies; no one needs to tell them how. It is not female sexuality that has a problem ('dysfunction') but society that has a problem in its definition of sex and the subordinate role that definition gives women.

Women find themselves in a state of 'sexual slavery' towards men, Hite claimed, providing them with sexual pleasure while ignoring their own needs. Equating the biological model developed by sexual science with the patriarchal oppression of women generally, she argued:

> The fact is that the role of women in sex, as in every other aspect in life, has been to serve the needs of others – men and children. And just as women did not recognize their oppression in a general sense until recently, just so sexual slavery has been an almost unconscious way of life for most women – based on what was said to be an eternally unchanging biological impulse. (...) Our model of sex and physical relations is culturally (not biologically) defined and can be redefined – or undefined.

In contrast, Hite drew on the social model of sexuality, arguing that:

> the pattern of sexual relations predominant in our culture exploits and oppresses women. It has institutionalized out any expression of women's sexual feelings except for those that support male needs.

Against this backdrop, Hite shifted the meaning of female lack of enthusiasm about sex from its traditional interpretation as the expression of sexual inhibitions from which women needed to be 'liberated', to a political act of 'resistance to participating in an institution which they have not had an equal part in creating', which was, in the report on male sexuality, explicitly compared to Gandhi's passive resistance of British rule in India.

Hite combated the 'sexual truths' produced by sexual science with its own weapons: legitimizing her claims by constantly referring to the authority of her 'scientific' data and methods. Her publications were nevertheless the target of bitter attacks from other sexologists such as Waldell Pomeroy, co-author of the *Kinsey Reports*, who questioned her methodology, 'political bias', and 'women's lib slant'; while feminists such as Jane Gallop criticized the 'science fantasy', that is, Hite's own emphasis on the scientific nature of her work, which, it was claimed, placed her necessarily in the same 'male place' as male sexologists.

Some feminists campaigned for the reform of the institution of heterosexuality, which was criticized for privileging male sexual needs, and called for better sex with men, naming the clitoris as a woman's new best friend. But others advanced 'political lesbianism' as an alternative. Following the American feminist Ti-Grace Atkinson's statement in the early 1970s that feminism is a theory, lesbianism the practice, authors such as Sheila Jeffreys, member of the Leeds Revolutionary Feminist Group, argued that women should exit relationships with men altogether, for as long as power relations between men and women remained unequal. Doing so, they believed, would foster relations of solidarity between women, though it would not require them to actually have sex with other women. As the Leeds group put it:

> We do think that all feminists can and should be political lesbians. Our definition of a political lesbian is a woman-identified woman who does not fuck men. It does not mean compulsory sexual activity with women.

Declaring lesbianism to be a matter of 'political choice' rather than a biologically determined sexual identity, political lesbians promoted a political version of the social model of sexuality. Sexual identity was not just defined by cultural, social, and historical context, they argued; it was a matter of voluntary political decision. As the Leeds group declared, since 'it is specifically through sexuality that the fundamental oppression, that of men over women, is maintained', political lesbianism was a crucial political strategy in the fight against patriarchy:

> Men are the enemy. Heterosexual women are collaborators with the enemy.

Authors such as Sheila Jeffreys and Adrienne Rich thus presented lesbianism as a position of resistance against patriarchy, one that did not need to include genital sex. Rich's 1980 essay 'Compulsory Heterosexuality and Lesbian Existence' advanced the concept of a 'lesbian continuum', according to which all women can share a 'range of woman-identified experience', from any form of 'bonding against male tyranny' to genital sex. Rich, in contrast to Jeffreys, did not ask heterosexual women to commit to lesbianism. The idea of a 'lesbian continuum' became an influential way of looking for points of solidarity between women in general, allowing for alliances between heterosexual and lesbian women.

In contrast, other voices within the women's movement argued for 'lesbian separatism', that is, the exclusion from women's lives not just of men, but also of heterosexual women. The latter, lesbian separatists argued, were guilty of collaboration through sleeping with men. As the most prominent lesbian separatist manifesto 'The Woman-Identified Woman', written in 1971 by the US collective Radicalesbians, put it: 'Our energies must flow towards our sisters, not backwards towards our oppressors.' Groups sprang up in most Western countries, such as Chicago Lesbian Liberation, Lesbian Separatist Group, Tribad, and

Collective Lesbian International Terrors in the United States, or the short-lived *Front des lesbiennes radicales* in France. They were, however, never more than extreme minority groups within the wider women's movement, and generated great hostility from other feminists who rejected the separatists' holier-than-thou attitude and 'phallic obsession', as Lynne Segal put it. In France, controversies around lesbian separatism led to the demise of the prominent feminist journal *Questions Féministes*, which had been founded in 1977 by an editors' collective that included Colette Capitan Peter, Christine Delphy, Emmanuèle de Lesseps, Nicole-Claude Mathieu, and Monique Plaza (later joined by figures such as Colette Guillaumin and Monique Wittig), under the directorship of Simone de Beauvoir. Whereas editors who left the journal argued that 'in the war of the sexes, hetero-feminism is class collaboration', when the journal was resuscitated as *Nouvelles Questions Féministes* in 1981, its editorial denounced lesbian separatism as 'terrorist' and 'totalitarian', 'incompatible with the principles of feminism', and emphasized that 'all women are oppressed by men as a class; ... feminism is the struggle against this *common* oppression'.

Feminist sex wars

Controversies over lesbian separatism also created tensions within the Women Against Pornography (WAP) group, whose founders in 1976 had included prominent figures such as Andrea Dworkin, Shere Hite, Gloria Steinem, and Adrienne Rich. Debates around pornography and prostitution, in turn, triggered major and bitter divisions among feminists, which became particularly intense during the 1980s. American organizations such as Women Against Violence Against Women, the UK Campaign Against Pornography, or New Zealand's Women Against Pornography defined prostitution and pornography as central to the oppression of women generally, in stark contrast to their portrayal within the sexual revolution as part of the wider march towards greater sexual liberation. Feminists such as Susan Brownmiller,

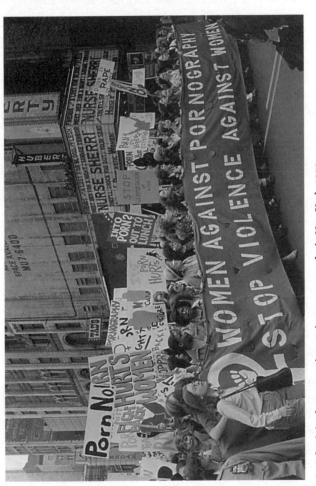

6. A feminist demonstration against pornography in New York, 1979

Andrea Dworkin, Catharine MacKinnon, and Susan Griffin conceptualized pornography and prostitution as forms of violence against women, and sexual violence as a key feature of male domination in general.

Controversially, they grounded their critique of female sexual exploitation in a broader analysis of male sexuality which identified violence as the underlying foundation of all male sexuality. As Brownmiller formulated it in her influential analysis of rape in 1975, *Against Our Will: Men, Women, and Rape*:

> From prehistoric times to the present, I believe, rape has played a critical function. It is nothing more or less than a conscious process of intimidation by which all men keep all women in a state of fear.

Rape, Brownmiller claimed, is a 'political crime against women', a weapon of patriarchy, as Kate Millett had also argued. Shere Hite agreed, stating in her report on male sexuality:

> Right now, forcible physical rape stands as an overwhelming metaphor for what has been the rape – physical, emotional and spiritual – of an entire gender by our culture.

From this perspective, pornography came to be seen as another manifestation of male violence against women, both during the production process of pornographic material, and in its consequences, by teaching men to eroticize the sexual subordination and abuse of women. Andrea Dworkin famously extended the analysis to intercourse itself, arguing that the sexual domination that she saw as central to pornography constitutes a basic feature of the ways in which men and women experience intercourse in patriarchal society. As she put it in 1987:

> In the fuck, the man expresses the geography of his dominance: her sex, her insides are part of his domain as a male. He can possess her as an individual – be her lord and master – and thus be expressing

a private right of ownership (the private right issuing from his
gender); or he can possess her by fucking her impersonally and thus
be expressing a collective right of ownership without masquerade
or manners.

Dworkin's views echoed statements made eight years earlier by the
Leeds Feminist Revolutionary Group, who had written:

Only in the system of oppression that is male supremacy does
the oppressor actually invade and colonise the interior of the
body of the oppressed. (...) Penetration is an act of great symbolic
significance by which the oppressor enters the body of the
oppressed.

Male sexuality was thus presented as intrinsically violent.
Whereas Dworkin located this violence within the historic context
of current gender relations, Catharine MacKinnon criticized
social-construction theories of sexuality for obscuring the
universal forms of the oppression of women through sexual abuse,
rape, prostitution, and pornography. The short-lived women's
collective Women Against Sex presented one possible conclusion
of such analyses when stating in the late 1980s:

There is no way out of the practice of sexuality except *out*... we
know of no exception to male supremacist sex... We name orgasm
as the epistemological mark of the sexual, and we therefore criticise
it too, as oppressive to women.

Not all feminists agreed, however. Critics such as Ellen Willis,
Gayle Rubin, Susie Bright, Lynne Segal, Carol Queen, and Carol
Vance began to define themselves as 'sex-positive' feminists,
in contrast to the perceived negative stance towards sex that
pervaded the anti-pornography and anti-prostitution crusades.
They attacked the anti-pornography stance on the grounds that
its analysis of porn, which made no distinction between violent,
misogynistic porn or porn produced for lesbians by lesbians, for

example, was over-simplistic; rejected the 'depressing' views of sex that reduce female sexual pleasure in intercourse to the result of male brainwashing; and denounced the dangers of the legal strategies pursued by anti-porn activists to freedom of speech in general, as well as the 'disturbing' political alliances with the religious Right (who meanwhile continued to combat women's and gay rights) the anti-porn crusaders had made.

In the US, organizations such as the Feminist Anti-Censorship Taskforce (FACT) were founded in the early 1980s to fight the attempts to legislate against pornographic materials led by Dworkin and MacKinnon; while the transnational feminist Global Alliance Against Traffic in Women, based in Thailand, combated the call for the abolition of all prostitution promoted by the US-based Coalition Against Trafficking in Women (CATW). The Alliance called for the decriminalization of voluntary prostitution, reconceptualized as a form of 'work' that women can choose to engage in, while battling against any type of forced prostitution and trafficking in women. Meanwhile, women working in the porn industry and prostitutes, who had recently started to found their own interest groups and trade unions, often vigorously objected against feminist labelling of their activities as inherently degrading for women (though the prominent porn star Linda Boreman, who had appeared in the notorious porn movie *Deep Throat* as 'Linda Lovelace', joined forces with MacKinnon and Dworkin). Adopting the 'sex work' label, organizations of sex workers argued that the political emphasis should be on trying to legalize and improve working conditions in the sex industry rather than trying to eradicate commercial sex altogether. Sex-positive feminism further spawned a series of thriving businesses, particularly in the US, specializing in the sale of women-friendly sex toys and publications, such as *Good Vibrations*, *Babeland*, the *Down There Press*, or the lesbian magazine *On Our Backs*.

The fights between 'sex-positive' and anti-prostitution/pornography feminists, described as the feminist 'sex wars'

7. Japanese sex toys, 1830

by Lisa Duggan and Nan Hunter, led to deep and permanent splits within feminism from the 1980s. One of the reasons for this is that the conflicts did not only concern differences about political strategies regarding commercial sex, but also involved fundamentally different ways of thinking about sexuality and its links to relations of power between the genders. In a context in which the women's movement came to be criticized by lesbians for privileging heterosexual concerns, by working-class women for reflecting middle-class interests, and by women of colour for being implicitly white, post-structuralist, postcolonial, and postmodern theories of gender emerged from the 1980s that rejected perceived simplistic binary oppositions between men-the-oppressors and women-the-passive-victims as politically mobilizing but conceptually unhelpful.

For example, as the African-American feminist Bell Hooks pointed out, sexual violence such as 'rape' has historically played a particularly important role for black women, as a central element of the system of slavery, and continues to impact on contemporary sexualized portrayals of black women; glossing over such differences in the name of universal male oppression is neither useful nor accurate. The category 'black feminist' has, in turn, also been criticized for masking cultural and class differences. For example, the African-American feminist novelist Alice Walker was actively involved in the international campaign against clitoridectomy, which is currently practised primarily in various countries on the African continent and some parts of the Middle East, as well as among some immigrant communities in Western countries. Feminist activists, including the prominent US feminists Gloria Steinem and Robin Morgan, joined third-world feminists such as the Egyptian Nawal El Saadawi to call for the redefinition of the practice as 'female genital mutilation' and a form of violence against women. As a result of international campaigns, the practice was declared a violation of human rights by Amnesty International and the United Nations, and made illegal in many Western as well as non-Western legislations since the mid-1990s. Whereas Alice Walker's earlier work had criticized white feminists for routinely excluding black women by speaking out on their behalf, her anti-female genital mutilation novel *Possessing the Secret of Joy* (1992), dedicated to 'the blameless vulva', and the documentary film *Warrior Marks* on the same topic which she co-produced, have been accused of cultural imperialism and neo-colonialism, for claiming to speak on behalf of African women on the grounds of her ancestry, while actually imposing an ethnocentric American vision of African cultural practices. More generally, Western feminists have been criticized for focusing on third-world cultural practices, while largely ignoring the fact that surgical interventions on women's genitals such as 'laser vaginal rejuvenation' and 'designer laser vaginoplasty' are currently among the fastest-growing areas of cosmetic surgery in many Western countries.

Whereas most feminists would promote a social rather than a biological understanding of gender identity and female sexuality, feminist thought on sexuality had primarily problematized female sexuality while treating male sexuality as, implicitly, unproblematic. Portrayals of male sexuality had echoed biological models of sexuality in taking for granted its naturally aggressive, triumphant, and, at times, violent nature. Feminist critics such as Lynne Segal, joined by theorists of masculinity – a field that greatly expanded in the 1990s – argued that it would be a mistake to conclude that this is also the way in which individual men experience sexuality. As Segal has pointed out:

> for many men it is precisely through sex that they experience their greatest uncertainties, dependence and deference in relation to women – in stark contrast, quite often, with their experience of authority and independence in the public world.

A significant degree of sexual anxiety, insecurity, and suffering on the part of individual heterosexual men, also emphasized in the work of Masters and Johnson, has been attested by empirical analyses of masculinity and male sexuality, including by feminist researchers such as Shere Hite, Wendy Hollway, or Susan Faludi. Whereas much of feminist theorization of sex has tended to equate heterosexuality with male domination, other feminist authors have thus emphasized the complexity of male and female sexual experiences. While not accepting male domination uncritically, they have stressed the need to take a closer look at what current transformations of masculinity mean for the dynamics of sexual interactions between men and women.

Feminist analyses of sexuality have constructed the institution of heterosexuality, the family, and intimate relationships as particularly important sites of the oppression of women by men, and therefore of political struggle. While this has led at least some radical feminists to argue for the abolition of the family (echoing the earlier views of Alexandra Kollontai or Wilhelm Reich), or the boycott of heterosexuality, the privileged focus on gender power within intimate relationships has also resulted in a comparative theoretical neglect of the role of state regulation of the family and sexuality. Paradoxically however, it is also in the context of the politics of sexuality that feminist activism has most frequently and successfully interpellated the state, albeit in contradictory ways. Whereas feminists have called for state legislation in areas such as rape, sexual harassment, and pornography, pushing these issues from the private into the public sphere, they have also argued against state intervention in matters such as abortion, on the grounds of a woman's 'private' right to decide. Feminist politics of sexuality have also, as we have seen, been the source of great conflict among feminists. Recent calls for more differentiated analyses of male and female sexuality have pointed out the importance of other types of identity, especially class and race, to the understanding of the ways in which power relations shape sexual experiences. As we shall see in the next chapter, gender, class, and race have also crucially shaped the regulation of sexuality by the state.

Chapter 4
The state in the bedroom

> The complex problems now confronting America as the result of the
> practice of reckless procreation are fast threatening to grow beyond
> human control. Everywhere we see poverty and large families going
> hand in hand. Those least fit to carry on the race are increasing
> most rapidly. People who cannot support their own offspring are
> encouraged by Church and State to produce large families. (...)
> Funds that should be used to raise the standard of our civilization
> are diverted to the maintenance of those who should never have
> been born.
>
> Margaret Sanger, c. 1921

The Aids crisis

The access to more reliable methods of contraception, the
legalization of abortion, and the relaxation of moral controls
on sexuality triggered by the sexual revolution opened up a
small window of greater openness, legal freedom, and sexual
experimentation from the 1960s which detached sexuality from
its traditional associations with sin and disease. The consequences
of these changes were profound, especially for women, for whom
sexuality had historically been entwined with the dangers of loss
of reputation, unwanted pregnancy, and death in childbirth.
In retrospect, the lighthearted celebration of greater sexual

opportunities – criticized by feminist thought for masking the exploitation of women by men – lasted less than two decades. The emergence of HIV/Aids (acquired immunodeficiency syndrome) from the early 1980s symbolized a move away from the hedonistic emphasis on sexuality as a site of pleasure. It revived earlier associations with danger and risk, echoing traditional anxieties about sexually transmitted disease, and about prostitutes and ethnic or racial 'others' as sources of sexual danger. It also set the stage for a return of religious models as major actors in the politics of sexuality.

The sociologist Jeffrey Weeks has argued that Aids revealed the unfinished character of the sexual revolution. On the one hand, sexuality remained primarily associated with heterosexuality not just within writings and therapeutic practices of sexologists such as Masters and Johnson and popular works such as *The Joy of Sex*, but also within areas of the feminist politicization of sexuality (as lesbian feminists had earlier complained). In this sense, the sexual revolution was a heterosexual revolution, as Sheila Jeffreys has pointed out. On the other hand, the loosening of moral control over sexuality, combined with the weakening of legal regulations against deviant sexualities, created societal conditions in which peripheral sexualities could flourish more publicly. The historically unprecedented growth in the West of lesbian and gay 'communities of choice' in the 1960s and 1970s publicly demonstrated the profound transformations of the sexual order that accompanied the sexual revolution and signalled a new era of political mobilizations around the rights of sexual minorities. Whereas lesbians and gays had been successful in establishing new public identities, the Aids crisis revealed, as Weeks contends, that traditional associations of homosexuality with disease and abnormality had not been suppressed irreversibly. With the advent of Aids, sexuality moved away from its connection with liberation to become once again fraught with anxieties and risks. As the American sexologist Theresa Crenshaw, president of the American Association of Sex Educators, Counselors, and

Therapists (AASECT), put it in 1987: 'the sexual revolution is over'.

Western responses to Aids were shaped by the political climate of the time. In countries such as the UK and the US, the 1980s saw the rise of the Right with the Thatcher and Reagan governments. The moral agenda of the Right was shaped in response to the claims of gay rights activists and the perceived threat from feminist critiques of dominant understandings of femininity and female sexuality. Whereas the sexual reforms of the 1960s had been promoted by the political Left, by the late 1980s, it was the Right which called for moral regeneration backed by state intervention. Particular targets were the 1960s liberalizations such as the legalization of abortion and homosexuality, as well as the greater legal freedoms in the areas of obscenity and censorship (attacks on the latter being supported as much by the moral Right as by certain strands of feminism that combated pornography).

The World Health Organization and UNAIDS currently estimate that more than 25 million people have died from Aids since it was first reported in Los Angeles by the US Center for Disease Control and Prevention on 5 June 1981, and that 38.6 million people presently live with the disease worldwide. A third of deaths from Aids have occurred in sub-Saharan Africa. While national rates of HIV infection currently exceed 20% in countries such as Botswana, Lesotho, Swaziland, and Zimbabwe, in some sub-regions over 70% of the population are estimated to be living with Aids. Such figures show the Aids pandemic to be one of the most destructive in human history. Since unprotected sexual contact is the main (though by no means only) vehicle of infection with HIV, Aids put sexually transmissible disease back at the forefront of collective anxieties about sex. As an infectious disease whose global spread was accelerated by long-distance trucking, mobile migrant work, tourist travel, and other forms of mobility characteristic of modern society, it required fast intervention both at the level of national states and at the international level. And yet, most governments were initially slow to react due to its initial identification as a disease that struck marginalized groups such as gay men, drug addicts, and ethnic minorities. Whereas 'innocent' victims such as haemophiliacs were to be pitied, the 'degenerate conduct' of promiscuous people meant that they were 'swirling around in a human cesspit of their own making', as the Chief Constable of Manchester, James Anderton, put it in 1988.

For the moral Right, Aids was the result of the permissive society. In the US, where the majority of Aids victims in the 1980s were black or of an ethnic minority, underlying racism further impacted on government inaction, and elsewhere the association of Aids with black people – in particular, Africans – or foreigners more generally structured public understandings of Aids as something brought in by 'outsiders'. Policies that were initially considered were primarily repressive in nature, including measures such as quarantine (supported by religious fundamentalists who saw Aids as divine retribution for immoral behaviour) or the mandatory testing of 'risk groups' and revival of anti-sodomy laws; measures that were promoted by conservative groups despite lack of evidence as to their effectiveness in curtailing the disease. Proposals for preventative sex education campaigns were treated with hostility from conservatives, who argued that they would encourage promiscuous behaviour. The first few years of the epidemic were furthermore characterized by recurrent media hysteria about the 'gay plague'.

Against the backdrop of governmental foot-dragging, most of the initial prevention effort in the West, especially in the UK and US, did not come from the state, but from grassroots organizations which had developed out of gay liberation and feminist movements. Voluntary organizations such as the Gay Men's Health Crisis (GMHC), founded in the US in 1981, or the Terrence Higgins Trust in the UK, set up primarily by gay activists, developed the concept of 'safe sex' and pioneered preventative sex education as well as support groups for people living with Aids, initially with minimal state support.

Gay organizations pursued different political tactics. For example, groups such as the GMHC centred on self-help, with the declared aim being the provision of care for the sick similar to that given by families or groups of friends – a crucial necessity in a social context in which biological families were often reluctant to assume that role themselves (reflecting the stigmatization of Aids and homosexuality in general). The GMHC's radical offshoot ACT UP – Aids Coalition to Unleash Power – campaigned for greater access to new drugs for people living with Aids. Adopting the slogan 'silence = death' and the pink triangle which the Nazis had used to identify homosexuals, they privileged shock tactics that aimed to publicly embarrass government officials into action. Other groups such as the Lambda Legal Defense Fund pursued the strategy of 'impact litigation' – consisting of the selection of cases not just for their impact on a particular person, but for the wider legal precedent that they would set – in areas such as discrimination in the workplace, aiming to improve the legal position of Aids sufferers as well as gays and lesbians more generally. The health emergency of Aids acted in turn as a further point of crystallization for political mobilization around gay rights. As Weeks has put it:

> The impact of the Aids crisis served to solidify the ties of community between gay people not despite but *because of* the threat it posed to their survival.

Sexologists were generally as slow to react to the emergence of the epidemic as governments. Deep internal divisions emerged over the most appropriate political response. In the US, for example, as the sociologist Janice Irvine reports in her analysis of modern American sexology, politically conservative sexologists such as Helen Singer Kaplan, Theresa Crenshaw, and Masters and Johnson rejected the notion of safe sex as a myth, and called for the 're-establishment of traditional values', to use Crenshaw's terms. Masters and Johnson's alarmist book *Crisis: Heterosexual Behavior in the Age of Aids* claimed in 1988 that Aids could be contracted from toilet seats and restaurant food (a claim that epidemiological experts strongly disavowed but which triggered a thriving commerce in 'anti-viral' toilet sprays). They called for mandatory testing of risk groups and for 'governmental crackdowns on prostitution'. Conservative American sexologists consequently frequently found themselves in political alliances with religious groups, as illustrated by Crenshaw's statement in 1987:

> I don't really mind if the right-wing leaders want to limit sexual practices to monogamy for religious reasons, if we want to limit them scientifically and the net result is the same.

Such positions were strongly rejected by other sexologists, however, many of whom became actively involved in the production of safe sex material and counselling.

Government responses to Aids

By the late 1980s, most Western governments had belatedly acquired a grasp of the urgent need for intervention, partly triggered by the rising numbers of heterosexual infections. The intensity of policy efforts varied across countries, however. Most Western countries introduced Aids-prevention measures in the form of poster and television campaigns and various forms of sex education from the late 1980s, and have repeated these since at varying intervals every few years. Switzerland had, in the mid-1980s and early 1990s, the highest level of HIV infection in Europe, partly due to relatively high levels of intravenous drug use. It is now recognized as the most proactive European country in publicizing Aids prevention, having introduced yearly nationwide Aids-prevention campaigns as well as a complete overhaul of its policies towards drug users, which have switched

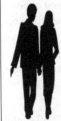

Lust, Sex, and Temptation
Are the normal sins of teenagers

<u>WE HAVE ALL SINNED AND BEEN FORGIVEN.</u>
JESUS TOLD US NOT TO CAST STONES.

Don't condemn our youth
to death from HIV/AIDS!

Provide both the Bible and condoms.

8. An example of an Aids-prevention poster campaign

from an emphasis on police repression to medicalization,
including free supply of sterilized needles; the result has been a
dramatic decrease in new cases of infection.

Debates continue, however, about which prevention policies
to promote, and have been the arena for major intervention
from religious models of sexuality. Controversies have centred
in particular on the promotion of condom use. Recognized by
medical experts to be the most effective protection against Aids
short of sexual abstinence, condoms continue to arouse great
opposition from fundamentalist groups and the Catholic Church,
who reject their interference with procreation and claim that they
encourage sexual promiscuity. The US and American-funded

programmes operating in developing countries currently privilege the ABC approach to Aids prevention, emphasizing 'Abstinence, Being faithful, and Condom use'. In the US and elsewhere, 'Just Say No!' campaigns promote sexual abstinence, while unmarried young people with a sexual past are encouraged to become 'born-again virgins' through a pledge to refrain from further sexual activity until marriage. However, such programmes have generally been unsuccessful in radically changing sexual behaviour or in reducing rates of HIV/Aids transmission, as health evaluations have demonstrated.

The emerging recognition that the majority of infections occur through unprotected heterosexual intercourse led to what has been described as a 'de-gaying' of Aids in the 1990s. Its results were received with ambivalence by gay activists. On the one hand, it was welcomed for decreasing the stigma associated with homosexuality. On the other hand, it meant that public funding, which had already been little forthcoming in the early years, was now not allocated with priority to gay support organizations, although gay men were still disproportionately affected by Aids. Some activists have consequently called for the 're-gaying' of Aids.

The issue of heterosexual infections with Aids also triggered further feminist critiques of sexuality. Building on the argument that Aids risk was not attached to certain types of people, as the focus on 'risk groups' had implicitly assumed, but to certain types of (unprotected) sexual practices, such as anal sex, feminist research such as the series of studies carried out in the early 1990s by Janet Holland and others explored the consequences of male sexual domination for risk-taking sexual behaviour. The research revealed that both heterosexual men and women tend to define and experience sexuality in relation to the primacy of male sexual 'needs'. Most partners adopt a biological understanding of male sexuality as the expression of natural, uncontrollable drives which should not be interrupted; a view which puts obvious constraints on women's possibilities for negotiating safer sex. Furthermore, normative female identity creates the dilemma for women that, on the one hand, contraception and Aids protection are seen as female responsibilities, while, on the other hand, women feel they should refrain from asking for anything that might spoil their partners' sexual pleasure. Interrupting the sexual performance of the male partner and being assertive about safety can run counter to being feminine, as Holland's team pointed out. The non-adoption of safer sex practices such as condom use does not, however, result from an external imposition of male power (at least not within the consensual relationships that were the focus of this study). As Holland's study demonstrates, male preferences are instead interiorized and actively reproduced by women, a mechanism the team describes as 'the male in the head'.

Various feminist analyses emerging from the area of Aids risk and prevention have thus been concerned with issues of women's power and powerlessness in heterosexual interactions, usually stressing the relative lack of power of women in sexual encounters with men. The reasons given for this powerlessness vary, however: different socialization for UK sociologist Janet Holland, economic dependency on men for Australian social psychologist Susan Kippax, or wider dominant definitions of heterosexuality for US anthropologist Carole Vance. Despite such divergent diagnostics, feminist research demonstrates the need to take gender identity into account when conceptualizing risk in sexual practices. Normative gender identities and gendered relations of power have clear implications for people's ability to prevent the sexual transmission of Aids; implications that government policies have in recent years attempted to try to build into their preventative strategies.

The health emergency created by Aids has constituted a major area for state intervention in citizens' sex lives, with sex education campaigns spelling out to them, in sometimes graphic detail, how they can avoid risk of infection with HIV. Initial government campaigns focused primarily on providing information as to how to prevent HIV infection, implicitly assuming that citizens were rational individuals who would abandon their risk-taking practices once they had been informed of their dangers. However, continuing new infections rapidly demonstrated that the provision of information, while crucial, did not suffice. Indeed, sexual interactions do not constitute the most rational area of most individuals' lives. In addition, we generally do not engage in sex as individuals, but in interactions with others, which again underlines issues of power and communication. The Aids crisis has thus demonstrated the importance for government prevention campaigns to take into account the emotional and irrational aspects of sex.

Eugenic 'race improvement'

Whereas state policies around Aids put the main emphasis on treatment, support, and transformation of sexual practices of individual citizens, other types of state action regarding sex have been primarily driven by collective concerns. At the collective level, sexuality carries particular symbolic importance, since it is through reproductive sexuality that the nation is biologically reproduced, which turns it into a concern of the state. As Michel Foucault put it:

> Sexuality has always been the site where the future of our species, and at the same time our truth as human subjects, are formed.

States have traditionally been preoccupied with the size and quality of their populations, concerns that have often reflected anxieties about the nation and its identity. Worries about decline in size or quality of the national population, about overpopulation, about 'surplus' of female or male children, or about whether immigrants are having more children than 'native' citizens have been recurrent items on national policy agendas. State concern with reproductive sexuality was particularly central to Western experiments with eugenics. The term 'eugenics' was popularized by Sir Francis Galton in 1883, to refer to the genetic improvement of the national 'stock' on the basis of the scientific study of 'all influences that tend, on however remote a degree, to give to the more suitable races or strains of blood a better chance of prevailing speedily over the less suitable than they otherwise would have had'. Galton regarded the evolutionary processes analysed by his cousin Charles Darwin, in particular the ideas of natural selection and the survival of the fittest, as too slow and uncertain for modern needs. Modern society put particularly high demands on its political elites, whose intellectual capacities were evolving too slowly, he argued. The 'science' of eugenics thus emerged during the second half of the 19th century, with the aim of assisting nation states in implementing social policies which would improve the quality of the national 'breed'. In opposition to the laissez-faire attitude of political liberalism, eugenicists advocated active social engineering. Individual citizens had a patriotic duty to contribute to the improvement of the nation through what Galton's successor Karl Pearson called 'a conscious race-culture'. As Havelock Ellis, a pioneer of both sexology and of eugenics, put it, 'sound breeding of the race' constituted 'our best hopes for the future of the world'.

Sexologists and psychiatrists were prominently represented within eugenic 'science' and activism. Eugenic thought in the first half of the 20th century comprised more precisely three central elements, which all reflected a profoundly biological model of human development: methods of selective breeding, worries about the physical and mental decline of the population, and ideas about the hereditary character of mental and physical illnesses and morally deviant behaviours – all of which directly affected ideas about sexuality and gender. As a combination of science and social movement, eugenics provided an analysis of what was wrong with modern society, how this occurred, and by what means it could be remedied. In the face of mounting threats and anxieties about 'degeneration', 'race suicide', and the threat of 'disorderly sexualities', eugenicists promoted a comprehensive programme of social engineering founded upon the rational management of reproductive sexuality by the state. It was to become an influential set of ideas, due to overlaps with other social and political concerns. Indeed, in the context of accelerating industrialization and urbanization processes, the rapidly growing urban population appeared as potentially destabilizing to the public order, while disciplined, healthy, and prolific citizens came to be seen as a source of wealth for expanding nation states.

The emergence of modern health and social policies from the turn of the 20th century provided the institutional conditions for translating eugenic rhetoric into a policy programme. Nowadays, eugenics tends to be popularly associated with Nazi Germany, where large-scale experiments in social engineering included forced sterilizations and 'euthanasia' of 'degenerate' persons. The 1933 Law for the Prevention of Hereditarily Diseased Offspring required doctors to register hereditary illnesses in their patients. In the course of the Nazi regime, over 200 'Hereditary Health Courts' were set up, which implemented over 400,000 sterilizations.

However, eugenic ideas found support across the political spectrum, including among socialists and anarchists. Social democrat reformers were among the pioneers of eugenic 'science' as well as policy practices in Europe. A number of eugenic policies such as forced sterilization of 'degenerates' were strongly promoted by the Left and pioneered in democratic countries. Socialist eugenicists placed great hope in eugenics as a social technology which could alleviate problems such as poverty and alcoholism, especially in combination with the eugenic education of citizens. Socialist versions of eugenics became part of the intellectual and political project of European social democracy. While feminists were to be found on both sides of the debate – supporting and opposing eugenics – most opposition came from liberals, who rejected state intervention in private life, and churches, particularly the Catholic Church.

Eugenicists called for scientifically founded state intervention to prevent further degeneration of the diseased national body. The emerging welfare state added an additional motive to that of preventing degeneracy: limiting public expenditure. Rapidly expanding welfare institutions increasingly targeted the 'inferior' categories of the national population, who became the main recipients of the growing welfare system. Limiting the number of 'weeds' in the national garden therefore appeared as a rational means of reducing welfare costs, which many social democrats as well as feminists supported enthusiastically. For example, Margaret Sanger, a prominent early 20th-century American feminist campaigner for sexual liberation and birth control – which would, she believed, liberate women from the biological burden of reproduction – was also an enthusiastic eugenicist. She wrote in 1925:

> Nature eliminates the weeds, but we turn them into parasites and allow them to reproduce.

Such 'human weeds' which 'clog up the path, drain up the energies and the resources of this little earth' should be eliminated from the national garden in order to 'clear the way for a better world', as she put it in 1922.

Eugenics offered the hope of a scientifically grounded elimination of all sorts of social ills and disorderly conduct, through policies that would carefully regulate the reproductive sexuality of the population. Other eugenic policies included education programmes, non-voluntary incarceration in psychiatric clinics, removal of children from parental homes, prohibition to marry, as well as measures that specifically targeted vagrants, 'gypsies', and, more generally, socially deviant groups such as unmarried mothers, 'sexual deviants', or people with physical or mental impairments. In Great Britain, eugenic preoccupations were clearly intertwined with the demands of the colonial empire, and much anxiety focused on the supposedly degenerative characteristics of the colonized, racial 'others' and the perils of interracial reproduction. However, despite widespread support for eugenics among leading intellectuals, the strong influence of liberalism in the UK, in particular the distrust of state intervention in private life, put a brake upon the translation of eugenic ideas into actual policy practice, at least at a national level. The political context was more favourable elsewhere in Europe. Countries such as Sweden and Switzerland – interestingly, neither of them colonial powers at the time – pioneered and applied eugenic policies to an extent that British eugenicists could only dream of.

Citizens' 'eugenic duties'

The eminent Swiss sexologist and socialist reformer Auguste Forel (1848–1931), Member of the Advisory Board of the International Federation of Eugenic Organisations and Honorary President of the World League of Sexual Reform in 1930, thus presented the construction of a social and national order based on the scientific management of reproduction by the welfare state as a moral duty to the future national community:

> The regulation of procreation through appropriate means is a moral task. It is necessary for the hygiene of our race. Only this, combined with the elimination of narcotic poisons, will be able to block the increasing degeneration of our race, and bring us a better future. We owe this to the progress, happiness and health of the future generations, for whose quality we are responsible.

Forel's view that the social order was based on hereditary dispositions and was under threat was combined with a traditional social-democratic belief in the redeeming powers of education. While 'only a healthy selection of the race' could improve the biological stock of the nation, this should be combined with active education campaigns based on science and reason:

> Let Science enlighten our sexual life freely and openly; then, the hypocrisy of normal people will cease, and that of abnormal people can be recognized in time and damage be prevented.

Given the importance of sexual selection for the regulation of procreation, Forel strongly promoted policies of sexual education. In his view, it was through selective, scientifically informed procreation that the boundaries around the national order were to be established and maintained. It was crucial, he argued, to teach young people about the consequences of having sexual relations with 'inferior' partners, and about the corresponding necessity of gathering information on the hereditary background of potential spouses. 'Each fiancée has the right and, in the interest of the future children, the holy duty,' Forel wrote, 'to know the sexual antecedents of their future spouse.'

In 1912, Switzerland prohibited marriage for the 'mentally deficient' and the 'legally irresponsible'. This made it the first European country to introduce a prohibitive marriage law based on eugenic rationale to prevent the reproduction of 'mental deficiencies'. Worldwide, the first eugenic sterilization law was introduced in Indiana in 1907, and by the 1930s almost two-thirds of US states had similar legislation targeting, in particular, institutionalized individuals such as criminals and those labelled 'mentally ill'. The notorious 1927 *Buck vs Bell* decision by the Supreme Court allowed the State of Virginia to sterilize a young single mother considered 'feeble-minded', who had been institutionalized to hide the fact that she had become pregnant from incest against her will, on the grounds that:

> It is better for all the world if, instead of waiting to execute degenerate offspring for crime or letting them starve for their

> imbecility, society can prevent those who are manifestly unfit from
> continuing their kind... three generations of imbeciles is enough.

In 1928, the Swiss canton of Vaud, influenced by Forel's ideas, adopted the first eugenic sterilization law in Europe. They were followed by Denmark in 1929, Germany in 1933, Sweden and Norway in 1934, and Finland in 1935. In the case of Switzerland, collective anxieties centred on the various social categories that were seen to constitute hereditary 'threats' to the Swiss nation: criminals, prostitutes, alcoholics, 'immoral' citizens (in particular unmarried mothers), the mentally ill, the physically disabled, haemophiliacs, people with tuberculosis, drug addicts, Jews, 'gypsies', and vagrants. It should be noted that the distinctions between labels such as sexual promiscuity, alcoholism, unsteadiness, dissoluteness, or 'squandermania' (a propensity for reckless spending) were often rather hazy. The 'mentally ill' were a particularly loose category which could include vagrants, people of 'weak morals', delinquents, and unmarried mothers (who were considered morally defective since they had clearly had sex outside of wedlock). Boundaries between medical diagnosis and moral values were, at best, fluid in eugenic discourse, and they completely dissolved in concepts such as 'moral feeble-mindedness'. Eugenicists such as Forel constantly called for the 'artificial sterilization' of the above-mentioned 'degenerate' categories of the population by the state, as a rational measure to prevent their reproduction. Forel perceived this task to be all the more urgent as he considered these sexualized 'others' and sexual 'perverts' – as well as women in general – as 'more sexual', and thus representing a particular reproductive threat to the nation.

Reflecting the eugenicist focus on female bodies as the reproducers of the nation, the sterilization of 'inferior' categories of the population was a strongly gendered practice. An early evaluation of the application of the Vaud law carried out in 1944 reported that nine out of ten eugenic sterilizations were carried out on women. Similarly, data from Zurich show that from 1929 to 1931, eugenic sterilizations were carried out on 480 women (in conjunction with abortion) and 15 men. Sterilization was also a heavily gendered practice in other countries: over 90% of the Swedish sterilizations were carried out on women.

The majority of legal sterilizations in the canton of Vaud – similar to the Swedish context – were applied to young, female social deviants, that is women who were deemed 'maladapted', living in poor conditions, mostly unmarried, and judged to have 'low intelligence'. The policing of respectable female sexuality appears to have been a central motive, since 'loose morals', 'uninhibited' female sexuality, or 'nymphomania', were frequently used as arguments for forced sterilization. In Zurich in the 1920s, for instance, prostitutes could legally be referred to psychiatric care when arrested. In a context in which 'feeble-mindedness' was considered to be more easily inherited by women than by men and prostitutes were considered to be particularly prone to pathologies, they were sometimes pressured into sterilizations. Sigwart Frank and Simon Jichlinksi, two psychiatrists who reported on sterilization practices in Switzerland in the 1920s and 1940s, provide extensive case stories exemplifying linkages between sexual transgressions and sterilizations. In 1931, the Directorate of the Poor Relief in Bern, the Swiss capital, issued a directive condemning the widespread practice of women's referrals for sterilization by welfare agencies and specifying that unmarried women, for instance, should only be sterilized 'if they show clear signs of physical or mental deficiency. [Sterilization] should henceforth not be carried out only because of sexual licentiousness if that person is otherwise physically and mentally normal.'

Sterilization could be applied against the consent of the person involved if she had been labelled as mentally defective. In other cases, methods for obtaining 'consent' included threatening withdrawal of welfare support or referral to a workhouse, or by granting permission to abort only on condition of simultaneous 'voluntary' sterilization.

Female bodies were a particular source of eugenic anxiety, as indicated by the gender imbalance in the removal of reproductive capacities. Reflecting traditional associations of reproduction with the female body, women were also seen as particularly important targets for the eugenic education and state regulation that eugenicists called for. As the sociologist Nira Yuval-Davis has pointed out, ideas about the 'purity of the race' tend to be crucially intertwined with the regulation of female sexuality. The prominent Swiss physician Imboden-Kaiser thus advocated an education programme that would instil in mothers a 'sense of reproductive responsibility', further developing Forel's principle of rational sexuality, while also calling for obligatory medical examinations and 'marriage ability attestations'.

While sterilization policies were the most extreme form of eugenic regulation of reproductive sexuality by the welfare state, these practices were complemented by 'preventative' education policies. The emphasis Forel and other campaigners placed on the necessity of eugenicist sexual education and marriage advice paved the way for the entrance of eugenics into the education curriculum. For example, an information brochure was produced and distributed in Swiss schools and officers' associations in 1939. The brochure educated Swiss youth about the dangers of reproducing with degenerate others, and pointed out their patriotic duty to the national collective. Youths were thus encouraged to:

> Choose your spouse from a physically and morally healthy, mentally superior family! You owe this to your offspring and to the Nation.

A Central Agency for Marriage and Sex Advice was set up by social-democrat welfare reformers in Zurich in 1932 – followed later by other Swiss cities – and organized exhibitions,

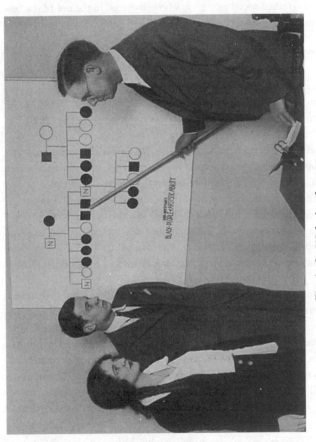

9. Eugenic marriage counselling in the US during the 1930s

presentations, and conferences on themes such as 'hereditary responsibility', 'psychiatric-eugenic advice on marital candidates' (1930s), and 'prevention of hereditarily diseased offspring' (1949). Sex and marital advice also constituted an area of political action for feminist social reformers who subscribed to the need for a 'less degenerate' future generation.

The notorious Swiss *Kinder der Landstrasse* ('Children of the Country Lanes') programme, a government-approved programme that aimed to eliminate vagrancy, had been set up by the federal child agency Pro Juventute and ran from 1926 to 1973. Its explicit aim was, in the words of its founding father Alfred Siegfried, to prevent the Yenish (the main group of 'gypsies' within Switzerland) from 'reproducing without restraint and bringing new generations of degenerate and abnormal children into the world'; it therefore sought the effective eradication of Yenish culture. In pursuit of these eugenic aims, Pro Juventute removed over 600 Yenish children from their parents, to be raised in orphanages, foster families, and mental institutions – an experience which a later prime minister, Ruth Dreifuss, described as 'one of the darkest chapters in modern Swiss history' in 1988.

Switzerland was by no means an exceptional case, however. It has been estimated that in Sweden, where eugenics was even more clearly intertwined with the construction of the social-democratic welfare state, 63,000 citizens were sterilized on eugenic grounds between 1934 and 1976. What is more, other European countries soon followed the Scandinavian and Swiss examples. Eugenic discourses were scientifically orthodox and their respectability was seldom questioned, and so eugenics seeped into mainstream culture in pre-Second World War Europe. The German Social Democrat Party (SPD), which had links with both the Swedish and the Swiss social democrats, played an important role in the development of left-wing versions of eugenics in the Weimar Republic, long before the Nazis applied a more radical form of eugenic policy. The SPD politicians Alfred Grotjahn (who also occupied the first Chair in Social Hygiene in Berlin) and Wolfgang Heine introduced the first eugenic measures, including the sterilization of disabled people, in the social-democratic-governed Prussia of the 1920s.

Social-democratic scientists, in particular sexologists, played as central a role in Germany as they did in Switzerland. For example, Magnus Hirschfeld was a prominent pioneer in the field of sexual reform and a homosexual himself. He was also a eugenicist who energetically campaigned against marriage for homosexuals. Indeed, he believed that, given their 'inferior' genes, homosexuals would be prone to giving birth to retarded children. Despite the fact that many social-democratic eugenicists, including Hirschfeld, later fell victim to the Nazis or fled Germany, they did not, as a rule, oppose Nazi measures such as forced sterilization, a practice that Hirschfeld considered 'an interesting experiment...', with the prudent qualification that 'it will be a long while before the results can be judged on their merits'.

Hirschfeld, like his friend and mentor Forel in Switzerland, was also involved with the social-democrat and eugenicist Marriage Advisory Board, which he had helped to develop in the context of his Institute for Sexual Science in the early 1930s and which became a forerunner of Nazi family eugenics. Disagreements with Nazi eugenicists centred, rather, on the 'fanatic' and consequently unscientific character of Nazi science, and especially on the matter of who should be included in the category of inferior persons. Indeed, social democrats such as Hirschfeld disapproved of the Nazi obsession with Jews (and complained that alcoholics and drug addicts consequently received less attention), a disapproval that was shared by British mainstream eugenicists. Interestingly, the *International Medical Bulletin*, which was edited in Prague by Jewish and social-democrat doctors who had fled Germany, attacked the 1933 Nazi sterilization law on political rather than ethical grounds: 'such a law is abused as an instrument of power in a capitalist state... only after a social revolution will it be possible to create the scientific and social conditions for "true" eugenics'.

In the UK and the US, a movement of 'Bolshevist Eugenics' emerged in the 1930s, which saw the Soviet Union as the only country that would be able to adopt a scientific stance towards the improvement of the community. In France, socialists such as Vacher de Lapouge, at various times a candidate for the *Parti Socialiste Ouvrier*, promoted the idea that citizens should fulfil a 'sexual service' in addition to their military service to the nation. Socialist versions of eugenics thus became part of the intellectual and political project of European social democracy. It is no surprise that social democrats were avid defenders of eugenics within the state as they held a firm belief in the responsibilities of the state towards its citizens, individually and collectively. As Forel put it, an 'intelligent, scientific (not dogmatic) social democracy' was needed in order to 'solve the eugenic problem'. In addition, social democrats promoted the subordination of individual interests to the collective good. Viewing eugenics as a social technology to alleviate poverty and social ills, social democrats conceptualized eugenic policies as being in the collective interest of the nation.

Although eugenic ideas were articulated from both sides of the political spectrum, and some social democrats strongly opposed them, social democracy nevertheless played a key role in the creation of eugenic technologies in countries such as Switzerland and Sweden between the 1930s and 1960s. It was within the framework of the axis of scientific disciplines, state actors, and private organizations that eugenic thinking was most 'successfully' applied, with social democrats being involved as civil servants, bureaucrats, and scientists. In Sweden and Switzerland, in the absence of the colonial encounter with other racial groups, preoccupations with racial purity turned inwards rather than outwards. This resulted in the intensifying categorization and hierarchization of 'internal others' such as 'gypsies', 'loose women', or the mentally and physically disabled, who were deemed to be sources of physical as well as moral degeneration. Policies were thus particularly engaged in the safeguarding of internal boundaries around the nation which had both a biological and a moral dimension.

It should be remembered, however, that there were internal divisions among social democrats regarding eugenics; moreover, social-democrat versions of eugenics were dwarfed by the Nazi programmes. It would be misleading to align social democracy and eugenics in any simplistic way.

The emergence of modern welfare policies and the presence of a favourable political context offered an institutional framework for attempts to realize the eugenic dream. Eugenic technologies such as sterilization without consent and marriage interdictions were combined with other measures such as eugenic education, sex education, and marriage advice. Limiting the numbers of those population categories that were to become the main recipients of the new welfare provisions appeared in this context as a rational means of cost reduction. Although not all policy-makers agreed with the eugenic emphasis on the influence of heredity rather than the social environment, the cost-reduction argument often led them nevertheless to support eugenically motivated sterilizations. After all, sterilization was a lot cheaper for the state than the long-term financial support of 'degenerates'.

The widescale social and political experiments with eugenics illustrate the concern of the state with the reproductive sexuality of its citizens. Drawing heavily on biological understandings, eugenic policies nevertheless failed to acknowledge the role played by men in reproduction. Politics around eugenics and Aids illustrates the complex intersections of sexuality with hierarchies around gender and 'race', and its connections to notions of individual and collective 'purity'. Both policy contexts suggest, moreover, that the interests of the individual do not always coincide with those of the majority. Collective mobilizations around state intervention in the area of sex have seen feminist and gay organizations occupy politically complex, and at times contradictory, positions.

Chapter 5
The future of sex

> The hesitantly speaking perverts of Krafft-Ebing's medico-forensic
> pages, confessing their most intimate secrets to the new sexual
> experts, have walked out of the clinical text and onto the stage of
> history, the living proof of sexual diversity.
>
> Jeffrey Weeks, 1986

Coalition politics

The 1960s and 1970s constituted a pivotal period of intensification
of public discussion and politicization of sex in the West, which
ultimately led to a fundamental review of the prevalent ways of
understanding and experiencing sexual practices and identities.
While the relaxing of moral and legal controls over sexual activity
is commonly taken to have been the defining feature of the sexual
revolution, feminist and gay critiques of the normative status of
heterosexuality have triggered transformations of sexual meanings
that are no less radical. Mainstream public discussion of sex,
however, remained at first firmly wedded to the idea that sexuality
meant – necessarily and only – heterosexuality. Typical popular
works of the time such as *The Joy of Sex*, which its author had
described as 'an unanxious account of the full range of human
sexuality', did not cover homosexuality or lesbianism, for example.
The similarly popular 1969 sex manual *Everything You Ever
Wanted to Know About Sex But Was Afraid to Ask* replied to the

question of 'what do female homosexuals do with each other?' as follows:

> Like their male counterparts, lesbians are handicapped by having only half the pieces in the anatomical jigsaw puzzle. Just as one penis plus one penis equals nothing, one vagina plus another vagina still equals zero.

And yet, the social and political changes of the time created a context that facilitated the greater public affirmation of 'peripheral' sexualities, to use Michel Foucault's term, most dramatically illustrated by the proliferation of lesbian and gay communities. Though pockets of same-sex subcultures, for example in the form of meeting places, can be identified earlier in modernity, particularly in large urban centres, the development of gay and lesbian cultural spaces and political organizations from the late 1960s onwards was unprecedented in human history.

The founding moment of the modern gay liberationist movement is commonly taken to be the spontaneous rebellion against a routine police raid at the Stonewall gay bar in New York in 1969, though many precursors existed, starting with the organizations defending the rights of sexual minorities that emerged in Germany towards the end of the 19th century around the exact same time the modern label 'homosexual' was invented. Stonewall was followed by the founding in 1969 of the National Gay Liberation organization in the US, the short-lived Gay Liberation Front in the UK in 1970, and many similar organizations in other countries. While some gay rights organizations, such as Lambda in the US, focused on reforming discriminatory policies from within existing political structures through litigation or lobbying strategies, others, such as the anti-hierarchical ACT UP, have pursued more unconventional and confrontational tactics towards the 'breeders' (heterosexuals). The unique problems posed by the appearance of Aids further galvanized political mobilization,

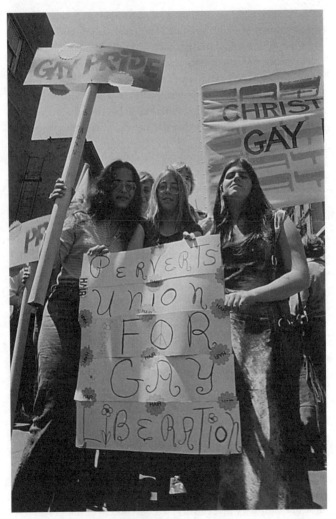

10. Gay liberation in New York, 1970

in particular of gay men. The sexual transmission of Aids, and the fact that it initially devastated large and already vocal gay communities in urban settings such as San Francisco and New York, helped to further unite gay men, strengthening collective identification with communities of choice both nationally and internationally. Many Western countries have subsequently passed a raft of gay rights legislation in crucial policy domains such as the military, employment, and civic partnerships, especially since the 1990s.

As part of their repertoire of political strategies, homosexuals have re-appropriated the labels that had been applied to them in the past, transforming their social meanings in the process. Terms such as 'fag', 'dyke', or 'queer', for example, initially used pejoratively, have been effectively co-opted by groups such as ACT UP and the New York organization Queer Nation, who adopted the defiant slogan 'we're queer, we're here' as an identity label around which gay pride and collective mobilization have been organized. In this vein, the use of 'gay' as a self-description, which spread from the American context in the 1950s and 1960s, marked the politicization of homosexual identity (leading to new identity divisions, as in 'he might be homosexual, but he's not gay'). More generally, many of the categories that 19th-century sexual science had so meticulously delineated, including transsexuals, transvestites, sadomasochists, paedophiles, and fetishists, have provided platforms for public self-affirmation and demands for recognition.

The increasing recognition of sexual diversity within politics, culture, the media, and the consumer industry has, in turn, led to a decline of the idea of 'perversion'. The sexological account of sexual normalcy that constructed the concept of the 'pervert' during the 19th century has been undermined by the public flowering of sexual minorities. As the sociologist Jeffrey Weeks puts it:

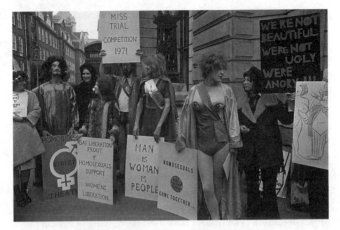

11. The Gay Liberation Front in London, 1971

> There no longer appears to be a great continent of normality
> surrounded by small islands of disorder. Instead we can now
> witness clusters of islands, great and small...New categories and
> erotic minorities have emerged. Older ones have experienced a
> process of subdivision as specialised tastes, specific aptitudes and
> needs become the basis for proliferating sexual identities.

The multiplication of identity labels has created difficulties,
however, for coalition politics around sexuality, forming a source
of possible tensions between respective political agendas. For
instance, while the interests of gay men and lesbians often
converge around issues such as parenting and adoption rights,
lesbians have questioned why they should focus activism on
Aids and sodomy laws (still in force in around 70 countries, but
usually enforced against male-to-male sex only) when such issues
have little impact on them. Lesbians perceive greater overlap
with the political agenda of heterosexual feminists rather than
gay men around health and reproductive policies, child care,
or discrimination against women in the workplace. Moreover,

some issues, such as the fight for improvement of breast cancer treatments, have been identified as affecting lesbian women particularly, since breast cancer disproportionately affects women who have not had children, which is the case for many (though by no means all) lesbians. Whereas many lesbian activists have strongly supported feminist campaigns for abortion rights, male gay organizations have generally refused to become involved with this topic on the grounds that 'it is not a gay issue'.

Furthermore, feminists, gay men, and lesbians have disagreed – both within and across these groups – over the respective merits of practices such as sadomasochism and pornography, while transsexuals and transvestites have been the object of feminist critique for perceived reinforcing of gender stereotypes. Feminists have also clashed with male gay activists over the promotion of 'gay marriage'. As the sociologist Stevi Jackson has pointed out, in the eyes of many feminists, the fight for gay marriage was about extending the male privilege anchored in the patriarchal institution of marriage to gay men and women, while leaving the gender hierarchy upon which the institution itself was founded – and which had led some feminists to call for the abolition of marriage in the past – unquestioned. Against this backdrop, some feminists, including lesbians, asserted that gay liberation had become a movement for male gay liberation. Thus political divisions between gay men and lesbians in the gay rights movement emerged in similar fashion to those, discussed in the previous chapter, between heterosexual and lesbian feminists.

Other sexual minorities created separate organizations. For example, and perhaps most controversially, paedophile interest groups emerged from the 1970s in numerous countries, including the Netherlands, the US, and the UK. Paedophile activism was particularly prominent in the Netherlands, where the respectable Dutch Sexual Reform Organization (NVSH) supported the publication in 1972 of the book *Sex met kinderen* ('Sex with Children'), which outlined international research on 'inter-generational sex', and which was widely drawn upon in paedophile political activism across Western Europe. In 1979, a petition to the Dutch Parliament calling for the legalization of consensual sexual relationships between children and adults was supported by the NVSH, feminist organizations, and the COC, the oldest still-existing gay rights organization in the world (founded in 1946). Around the same time, the Protestant Foundation for Sex Education (PSVG) distributed tens of thousands of copies of an information booklet with the title *Paedophilia* to Dutch elementary schools (1979–81).

In contrast to the World Health Organization's characterization of paedophilia as a sexual and mental disorder, paedophile activists argued for greater legitimacy, declassification of paedophilia as mental illness, children's sexual rights, and the decriminalization of (consensual) inter-generational sex. In France, various public petitions of the late 1970s called on Parliament to abolish age of consent laws; in particular, a 1977 petition calling for the decriminalization of all consenting relations between adults and minors was signed by prominent public intellectuals including Jean-Paul Sartre, Simone de Beauvoir, Michel Foucault, Jacques Derrida, Roland Barthes, and France's most prominent child psychoanalyst Françoise Dolto. Paedophile advocacy groups thus operated in a context in which cultural ideas about children's sexuality were being redefined more generally, and in which the age of sexual maturity had dropped significantly, probably due to better health and nutrition. For example, by the 1960s to 1970s, girls reached puberty on average around the age of 13 in Western countries, as well as among prosperous groups in many non-Western countries, compared to 16 or 17 a century earlier; and boys reached physical sexual maturity around 17, compared to 23 in the mid-19th century; a trend that has continued since.

Groups such as the Paedophile Information Exchange (PIE) in the UK (created in 1974); North American Man Boy Love Association

(NAMBLA) in the US (created in 1978); the Danish Paedophile Association (DPA) (set up in 1985); and International Paedophile and Child Emancipation (IPCE) (founded in the early 1990s), drew on Freudian theories and on sexological research, including the Kinsey Reports, to argue that children are sexual beings, and on ancient Greek models of sex to argue for the 'educational benefits' of such relationships.

While always a controversial issue among the wider population, public attitudes towards adult–child sexual relationships have hardened significantly since the 1980s, though important cultural variations remain. In Western Europe, paedophile political lobbies have mostly withered away in the face of increasing public outrage at sexual abuse of children, and although in the Netherlands a 'Love Thy Neighbour, Freedom and Diversity' Party was founded in 2006 whose aims included seeking to decriminalize sexual activities at any age unless they are dangerous or coerced (it also supported the criminalization of sexual maltreatment of animals, currently not punishable in Dutch law), it was unable to raise the required number of public signatures from Dutch citizens to participate in actual elections. In the US, Canada, and the UK, increasing police surveillance and criminalization of their members have led many – though not all – of the most prominent groups to disband or to transform into less visible Internet-based communities.

Political alliances initially existed between paedophile groups and some gay rights organizations, for example around issues such as the age of consent (the minimum legal age at which individuals are considered to be capable of giving informed consent to sexual relations). The legal age of consent is currently set around 17 or 18 in many countries, with limits of 12 in the Philippines, 13 in Spain and Japan, and 14 in Germany and Italy at the lower end of the scale. Sex outside of marriage is illegal at any age in countries such as Saudi Arabia, Pakistan, and Iran. Age of consent legislation constituted a major issue of gay rights mobilization over the past few decades, since in many countries the age of consent for sexual relations between men was set higher than that for heterosexual relations or same-sex relations between women (which were less commonly criminalized), though many countries have equalized the age of consent in recent years. In contrast, around 70 countries currently criminalize homosexuality (and, in the case of Zimbabwe, same-sex hand-holding as well) altogether.

Gay rights organizations' alliances with paedophile activism around the age of consent issue, or more generally on the grounds of solidarity with other sexual minorities, have melted away since the early 1980s. In large part this was the result of campaigns from the Christian Right such as the US conservative activist Anita Bryant's self-proclaimed 'crusade' against 'the threat of homosexual recruitment of our children', entitled *Save Our Children*, which portrayed all gays – and gay men in particular – as potential child molesters and triggered the start of organized opposition to gay rights organizations in the US from the late 1970s. While the Dutch gay rights organization COC had declared in the early 1970s that gay liberation would never be complete without the sexual liberation of children and paedophiles, by the mid-1990s the great majority of gay rights organizations had distanced themselves explicitly from paedophile advocacy and condemned the campaigns for the removal of legal protections against sex between adults and children as sexual abuse, as illustrated in the statement about NAMBLA from a representative of the Human Rights Campaign, the largest US lesbian and gay lobbying group: 'they are not part of our community and we thoroughly reject their efforts to insinuate that paedophilia is an issue related to gay and lesbian civil rights'.

In other policy areas away from paedophilia, strategic alliances were successfully formed. Attempts at greater inclusiveness and coalition politics between different sexual minorities are symbolized by the currently prevalent umbrella label 'LGBT' (Lesbian, Gay, Bisexual, and Transgendered community). This already precarious wider grouping has come under attack, however, from black homosexual activists, who have argued that concerns over black homophobia have been privileged over addressing hidden racism within gay rights organizations. Despite the influence of the black civil rights movement in the US on gay political mobilization, the importance of cultural icons such as Bessie Smith and Audre Lorde, and the prominent role black homosexuals and transvestites played in the context of the Stonewall Rebellion and political responses to Aids, black gays and lesbians are, they feel, underrepresented among the leadership of gay rights organizations and their specific concerns are insufficiently included on gay political agendas.

Sexual separatism

Sexuality

Disagreements as to whether to focus efforts through 'single-issue' organizations or to pursue much broader aims have also given rise to separatist strategies. Indeed, this has been a recurring theme since the early days of homosexual activism. The very first movements for the rights of sexual minorities which arose in Germany around the turn of the 20th century were already split around this question, with the Scientific-Humanitarian Committee (1897), led by the sexologist Magnus Hirschfeld and based upon a 'third-sex' model of homosexuality, tending towards a gay-separatist model of alliances between gay men and lesbian women, while the *Gemeinschaft der Eigenen* ('Community of Self-Owners'), co-founded in 1902 by the anarchist Adolf Brand, the sexologist Benedict Friedlaender, and the youth movement activist Wilhelm Jansen, promoted a gender-separatist model of alliances between gay and heterosexual men. The Daughters of Bilitis, generally recognized as the first organization for lesbian rights, founded in San Francisco in 1955, broke apart in the 1970s over internal disagreements regarding the prioritizing of commitment to women's rights over specifically lesbian interests. Furthermore, the American National Organization of Women (NOW) called for the expulsion of the 'lavender menace' from its ranks, fearing that vocal lesbian presence would increase media hostility towards the movement.

Some strands of lesbian separatism of the 1970s and 1980s radicalized such controversies in seeking not only organizational, but also geographical, independence. Most prominently, Jill Johnson's 1973 work *Lesbian Nation: The Feminist Solution* argued for 'tribal groupings' of 'the fugitive Lesbian Nation', calling for separate lesbian social and cultural spaces which could act as a power base within the wider women's movement. Dutch radical-feminist groups dreamt in the early 1970s of establishing an independent lesbian community on a 'women's island', a utopian idea that was echoed when Australian activists declared the small islands of Cato to be the new micro-nation Gay and Lesbian Kingdom of the Coral Sea in 2004, issuing its first postal stamps in 2006. Territorial separation of either lesbian-only or women-only groups was achieved – if only temporarily – with the founding of women-only spaces and festivals with names such as 'herland', 'wimminsland', and 'Womyn's Festival' in the US, Canada, and Australia, satirized in Armistead Maupin's *Tales of the City* novels. Territorialized strategies were revived by the US radical feminist Dworkin's call, in 2000, for a separate homeland for women. Male gay authors such as William S. Burroughs have similarly called for a gay nation state, and organizations such as the German-based Gay Homeland Foundation, created in 2005, aim to persuade 'the government of a large and thinly-populated nation' to sell a stretch of 'uninhabited land' where an independent state would be established for lesbian, gay, bisexual, transsexual, and transgendered citizens.

Virtual versions of separatism around gender or sexual identity are incarnated in the recent writings of the British 'Miss Martindale', the self-proclaimed public face of 'the feminine empire Aristasia' where men do not exist and the two sexes are 'blonde' and 'brunette'. Semi-religious versions of separatism emerged from the 1980s in the shape of spiritual organizations across the world such as the Re-formed Congregation of the Goddess International, and Dianic Paganism, some types of which have been associated with lesbian separatism. The latter, following Zsusanna Budapest's 1975 'ovarian book' *The Holy Book of Women's Mysteries*, regroups 'neo-pagan feminist goddess-worshippers' in Wiccan groups or in non-Wiccan covens which draw heavily on biological models of femininity to celebrate female reproductive powers, women's bodies more generally, 'womanism', and 'the divine feminine'.

The territorialization of sexual and gender politics involved different activist strategies for radical groups such as Queer Nation, which emerged in New York in 1990 and produced the deeply controversial slogan 'I Hate Straights'. Queer Nation epitomizes newer approaches to the politics of sexuality in no longer demanding the right to sexual freedom in the privacy of the home, or in literally separate 'homelands', but instead calling for the de-heterosexualization of the public sphere through actions such as 'queer nights out' in straight clubs by groups like the Lesbian Avengers. Being queer is, they argue, not about the right to privacy, but about the freedom to be public. Whereas separatist political lesbianism promoted 'fugitive' exit from the heterosexual colonizer, the new cultural (rather than ethnic) nationalism of queer nationalism calls for the gay re-colonization of public spaces by eradicating heterosexist homophobia.

In theoretical terms, queer theory, as associated with authors such as Judith Butler, Eve Sedgwick, Teresa de Lauretis, Michael Warner, and Steven Seidman, and developed from the early 1990s onwards, has built upon earlier radical feminist theorization and critique of normative heterosexuality by Adrienne Rich, Monique Wittig, and others. Queer theory emphasizes the socially constructed nature of gay and lesbian categories, echoing the earlier writings of Michel Foucault, symbolic interactionist sociologists such as Gagnon and Simon, Ken Plummer and Jeffrey Weeks, and theorists of political lesbianism. Though the term 'queer' encapsulates a plurality of meanings, it primarily refers to the rejection of binary categorizations such as man/woman and gay/straight. Instead, the multiplicity and instability of identity labels in general is emphasized. As the sociologist Diane Richardson puts it:

> We are, it is suggested, post such identities: post woman, post man we are transgender; post lesbian, post gay, post heterosexual (perhaps?) we are queer.

Culturally, queer theory involves an emphasis on 'permanent rebellion' and subversion of dominant social meanings and identities. For some authors, this includes a vehement rejection of the spectacular development of gay consumer culture since the 1980s, including gay travel agencies, bars, bathhouses, legal services, therapists, and fashion outlets, as expressed in the slogan 'we're here, we're queer, and we're NOT going shopping'. Instead of promoting assimilation into mainstream society, queer theory aims radically to transform the social order by destabilizing not only the taken-for-grantedness of heterosexual norms, but also stable, biologized understandings of gay and lesbian identity as well as gender. Gender and sexual identities are, it is argued, fluid and unstable, as queer author Kate Bornstein illustrates when describing herself in the following terms:

> In a nutshell, I used to be a het guy who did the gender-change thing and became a grrl, a lesbian grrl at that. Then, after my female lover became a guy, I stopped calling myself a lesbian. Being a lesbian had become too complicated. Calling myself a lesbian managed to offend just about everyone, so I began to call myself a dyke.

The US sexologist Carol Queen and novelist Lawrence Schimel coined the term 'PoMosexuals' in 1997 to describe 'POst-MOdern' individuals such as Kate Bornstein, who graphically illustrate the fluid nature of both gender and sexual identity. In their words:

> We pomosexuals are the queer's queers, the ones who will not stay
> in the boxes marked 'gay' and 'lesbian' without causing a fuss – just
> as we all burst out of the boxes the straight world tried to grow
> us in.

Pomosexuals, the 'bastard children' of the gay and lesbian
movement, as the American self-identified 'troublemaker' and
'S/M writer of gay male pornography for women' Pat Califia puts
it, break the intricate links between gender and sexuality involved
in the labels gay, lesbian, and heterosexual.

Politically, queer activism – numerically a very small movement –
involves an emphasis on inclusiveness and solidarities around
diversity. Queer politics has also, however, involved calls for
a renewing of alliances between lesbians and gay men on the
grounds of the prioritization of common identities as 'queers' over
that as women. Some versions of queer political theory criticize
gay and lesbian organizations for implicitly assuming homosexual
identity as unified and stable. Similarly, radical feminism has
been attacked for naturalizing the category of 'woman' (as well
as for its presumed 'moralistic' stance). In contrast, in a queer
future, sexual labels such as gay, lesbian, as well as heterosexual,
would be subsumed in the overarching fluid identity of queer,
as is argued by queer theorists, who often prefer to speak of
LGBT&F (Lesbian, Gay, Bisexual, Transgendered, *and Friends*).
The current reality is, however, different, as the writer D. Travers
Scott put it:

> Queer almost immediately came to mean 'saucy fags and dykes',
> not the radically-sexualised boundary-breaking coalition it was
> first advertised to be, or we'd have a hell of a lot more heterosexual
> 'queers' in our parades.

Moreover, the privileging of solidarities across different identity
labels has led to criticisms of a 'false unity' which glosses over
specific discriminations around gender and race. Judith Butler,

seen as one of the most prominent queer theorists, has raised such questions in her own writings, while also warning against the idea that feminism and queer theory are somehow incompatible.

Queer theory echoed earlier criticism of sexual liberation, including gay liberation, politics (or the sexual liberation promoted by Reich and Marcuse) by Michel Foucault, who famously rejected the implicit assumption of liberationism that there was such a thing as a natural, biological sexuality that could be 'liberated'. As Foucault and other social constructionists emphasize, sexuality should instead be viewed as a social experience that is shaped by its social and political context. However, while political mobilization based upon tactics such as 'coming out' and 'outing' (declaring public figures to be gay) have, on the one hand, solidified the categories of gay and lesbian, the emphasis on sexual identity as 'choice' and political practice (though not shared by all gay activists) also denaturalizes sexual identity. Moreover, the wider categories of gay and lesbian have been the object of greater fragmentation since the time of Foucault's writings, as reflected in commercial and activist subcultures which cater for leather dykes, S/M gays, butch/fem lesbians, denim queens, lipstick lesbians, bisexuals, pan- or omnisexuals, gay Republicans, anarcho-lesbian-feminists, gay veterans, gay Mormons, British gay skinheads, or Daddies (older gay men with a sexual interest in young, adult men). Both the denaturalization and the fragmentation of wider identity labels and related political interests serve to create new opportunities for sexual politics, as well as new difficulties for coalition politics and new exclusions.

Conservative sexual politics

Radically social models of sex as promoted by queer theorists and embodied by pomosexuals have competed with a major revival of both religious and biological models of sexuality over the past two decades. The Catholic Church, for example, still officially defines homosexuality as a 'moral evil'. The rise of Christian and other religious fundamentalisms throughout the West from the 1980s has reinvigorated traditional moral condemnations of sexual deviancy. In the political arena, the activism of the Christian Right has generally been the source of the most vehement opposition to gay rights campaigns, especially in America. As a social movement, the Christian Right draws primarily from Evangelical Protestant groups which aim to defend and restore 'traditional values' against the 'moral decay' of the rise in sexual permissiveness, and perceived threats to the patriarchal, heterosexual family resulting from feminism and gay rights campaigns.

Political strategies differ within the movement, however. Mass movements such as the Promise Keepers, an American Christian men's movement, focus on a commitment to 'spiritual, moral ethical, and sexual purity' (promise 3) and to 'building strong marriages and families through love, protection and biblical values' (promise 4), but prioritize a focus on masculinity rather than on sexual orientation – which is indirectly present in their primary aim of restoring the traditional gender role of men within the heterosexual family. In contrast, American organizations such as the Traditional Values Coalition tend to see gays not only as immoral, but also as out to undermine society and 'recruit' the young, and they consequently specialize in the fight against gay rights. The notorious Westboro Baptist Church in Kansas welcomes various ills that befall America, including Aids, 9/11, and the death of US soldiers in Iraq, as well-deserved punishments from God for America's tolerance of homosexuality. On its website 'God Hates Fags' (opening words: 'welcome, depraved sons and daughters of Adam'), it argues that 'God Hates America' (as well as Sweden, Canada, Ireland, and Mexico) for its 'Godless sodomite culture'.

Many Western countries have Christian support groups for gay men and women that depict homosexuality as a misguided lifestyle choice, and undertake to 'help' those who wish to lead a 'proper' heterosexual lifestyle. Among the largest of these, EXODUS International, for example, promises 'freedom from homosexuality through the power of Jesus Christ', offering 'reparative therapy' to 'men and women who struggle with unwanted homosexual attractions' and who want to 'grow into heterosexuality', as well as annual international 'freedom conferences' (the 2007 conference was titled 'Revolution').

Although religious and conservative groups that reject sexual diversity in the name of 'family values' have largely monopolized moral models of sexuality, alternatives founded on respect for sexual pluralism are, of course, implicit in equal rights campaigns. Faced with recurring moral fundamentalisms and sexual conservatisms, authors such as Jeffrey Weeks and various queer theorists have attempted to elaborate alternative, 'progressive' value models for sexuality. Furthermore, liberal theologians from various religious affiliations have vocally supported gay rights claims, drawing on different versions of Christian ethics, while neo-conservative redefinitions of sexual identity promote equality from a political standpoint which is both conservative and libertarian in contrast to the Left-activist position that forms the basis for queer politics. This type of counter-queer gay politics is personified by Andrew Sullivan, the British author of *The Conservative Soul: How We Lost It, How to Get It Back* (2006) who lives in America, or by the Log Cabin Republicans (the gay wing of the Republican Party); while on the cultural plain, the 'Bears' movement, which celebrates conventionally masculine-looking gay or bisexual men with hairy bodies and facial hair, and rejects what it perceives as 'effeminate' styles and mannerisms, has been gathering steam in recent years.

Biological models of sexuality have been reinvigorated by the recent expansion of evolutionary and genetic science, as exemplified in the ambitious Human Genome Project which has undertaken to map the entire sequence of human DNA.

Developments in genetic research have repopularized biological and hereditary understandings of sexual practices and identities. For example, beliefs that homosexuality could be explained by a 'gay gene' were triggered by a study by Hamer and others on fruit flies, published in *Science* in 1993, which claimed a link between genetic make-up and sexual orientation – a finding that has since been heavily contested. Various 1990s studies have attempted to identify specific biological characteristics such as more frequent left-handedness in gays, while other studies continue to argue that homosexuality is caused by a disorder in sex hormones. Institutions such as the American Department of Defense continue to define homosexuality in biological, medicalized terms, as a mental disorder. Finally, the pharmaceutic development of potency products such as Viagra further involves the profound medicalization of sexuality.

Biological models of sexuality have been adopted to legitimize opposing positions within the politics of sexuality. For example, on the one hand, the claimed discovery of a 'gay gene' has led to calls for genetic 'correction' of sexual deviancy. On the other hand, a representative of Lambda welcomed the 'discovery' of the gay gene in *Time Magazine* in 1993 on the grounds that such a finding meant that homosexuals 'can't help the way they are' and should therefore not be discriminated against. Just like religious models, biological understandings of sexuality have served both to pathologize sexual deviancy and to sustain equal rights claims.

Recent developments in the area of genetics have also revived collective preoccupations with heredity, reproductive control, and the future of welfare systems, and returned such issues to the political agenda. New practices such as genetic counselling during pregnancies have led to misgivings based upon past eugenic experiences for some, and triggered new hopes for improvement of the collective genetic stock of the nation for others. For example, the genetic scientist Herman Muller set up a 'sperm bank' in the US which operated until 1999 and was intended to raise the genetic 'quality' of America by providing sperm from Nobel prize laureates, an aim that failed miserably due both to the reluctance of the intended donors to get involved and the low quality of the sperm of those few (elderly) scientists who did.

More generally, concerns with higher levels of reproduction from what are regarded as 'undesirable' categories of citizens, such as Muslim immigrants, were publicly articulated by politicians in countries such as France in the 1990s, echoing older Western worries about fertility levels in non-Western countries such as India and China. Female reproductive sexuality continues to constitute a particular policy concern of the state. For example, in America in the early 1970s, an estimated 100,000 to 150,000 women on low incomes were sterilized annually under federally funded programmes, frequently under the threat of withdrawal of welfare benefits. Following action from the US Committee to End Sterilization Abuse, a federal judge put an end to the legality of such practices in a 1974 ruling, but it is generally recognized that this failed to put a halt to coerced sterilization. By the early 1980s, an estimated 24% of African-American women, 35% of Puerto-Rican women, and 42% of American-Indian women (compared to 15% of white women) had been sterilized, many of them without their consent or full understanding of the consequences. Current organizations such as Project Prevention/CRACK ('Children Requiring A Caring Kommunity') offer cash incentives to male and female drug addicts who accept sterilization or vasectomy, and Republican politicians have triggered accusations of 'neo-eugenics' by calling for forced sterilization of 'disorderly' categories of the population, including crack-addicted mothers and other welfare recipients, since the 1990s.

In European countries, recent cultural battles around immigration have centred on controversies around sexual ethics. Muslim immigrants, in particular, are accused of rejecting both Western sexual liberation and women's liberation, and of lack of tolerance

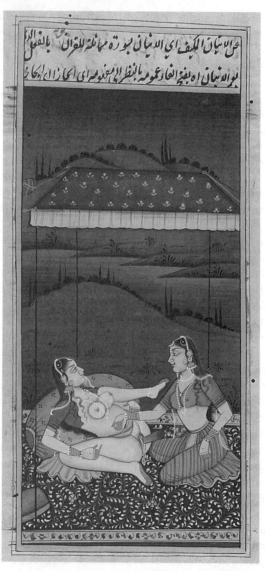

12. A woman caresses another woman, who uses a root vegetable as a dildo, 19th century, India

towards sexual diversity. The portrayal of cultural 'outsiders' as more sexually repressed than the native population is an interesting reversal of earlier historical depictions of non-Western sexuality. Indeed, 'Oriental' cultures have traditionally been the repository of Western sexual fantasy. Exotic representations of 'the Orient' which conjured up images of Eastern unlimited sensuality and guilt-free licentiousness have been a persistent theme among Western intellectuals, including the 18th-century French political theorist Montesquieu in his *Persian Letters* (1721), 19th-century French novelist Gustave Flaubert, or the 19th-century British explorer Sir Richard Burton (translator of *Arabian Nights* and the *Kama Sutra*). In a similar vein, early Western anthropologists such as Margaret Mead in *Coming of Age in Samoa: A Psychological Study of Primitive Youth for Western Civilization* (1928), or Bronislaw Malinowski in *The Sexual Life of Savages* (1929), have routinely portrayed non-white races as closer to nature and therefore much freer sexually, in contrast to the more civilized, and therefore sexually more restrained, West. Cultural stereotypes of black men as sexually potent and better-endowed than white men further reflect the projection of Western sexual as well as racial fantasies and anxieties.

Sexuality and power

Recent controversies around sexuality thus further illustrate the intricate links between sexuality and the social relations of power flowing from gender, social class, and 'race' that have, historically, shaped it. As Michel Foucault put it, sexuality constitutes

> an especially dense transfer point for relations of power: between men and women, young people and old people, parents and offspring, teachers and students, priests and laity, an administration and a population.

Contrary to the sexual liberation paradigm, sexuality cannot, in this view, simply be pitted against power. As we have seen,

Freudian Marxists such as Marcuse, Reich, or Fromm argued in the 1960s that sex is a positive force which is repressed by modern civilization and capitalism, and that sexual liberation will transform the social order. Such hopes that the sexual revolution would not only liberate sexuality but also subvert wider repressive structures of power have faded since.

But the connections between sexuality and power are all the more important because our relation to ourselves as sexual beings constitutes such a central component of modern identity, as Foucault emphasized. A similar point is made by the British sociologist Anthony Giddens, who argues: 'Somehow ... sexuality functions as a malleable feature of self, a prime connecting point between body, self-identity, and social norms.' The two authors disagree, however, on the political implications of the centrality of sexuality to modern self-identity. Whereas for Foucault, sexuality is a prime target of modern relations of power and fundamental to processes of societal disciplinarization of 'disorderly' populations, Giddens identifies the spread of the 'pure' relationship over the past few decades as a positive phenomenon; by 'pure' relationships, he means to denote a type of relationship which, in a social context where women's economic dependency towards men has lessened and exit options such as divorce have become accessible on demand, exists for its own sake. Though more fragile than traditional marriage, which was propped up more firmly by wider social institutions, the pure relationship involves transformations of intimacy that contribute towards a democratization of the private as well as the public sphere. Concentrating on heterosexual relationships, Giddens, as well as the German sociologists Beck and Beck-Gernsheim, see women as the vanguard of more equal understandings of sexuality and intimacy. In their view, transformations of male sexuality are largely a result of women's struggles to change their lives. As Beck and Beck-Gernsheim put it: 'men's liberation is a passive affair'. Men, they add, 'seem to engage in self-liberation as spectators'.

Certainly, relations of power between men and women have shifted dramatically over the past few decades, as have normative models of femininity and masculinity. Whereas male sexuality has been theorized as inherently violent, alternative accounts have emphasized the passivity and vulnerability of male (hetero-)sexual experience, against the backdrop of a wider 'crisis of masculinity' to which groups such as the Promise Keepers provide a fundamentalist answer. Similarly, recent controversies over the potency drug Viagra could be read in different ways: the speed of its availability on the market could be seen as a sign of the triumph of male wishes or, alternatively, as further contributing to the myth (and psychological pressure) of unproblematic male sexual performance. In terms of intersections between gender and sexuality, analyses have currently come full circle, from the pathologization of female sexuality and taken-for-grantedness of male heterosexuality as the norm within sexual science and medicine, to greater problematization of male sexual experience, reminding us, in the words of the political theorist Terrell Carver, that 'gender is not a synonym for women'.

Since the late 1980s, sexuality has figured prominently on Western political agendas, covering national as well as international issues. Controversies around teenage pregnancy rates, prevention of sexually transmitted disease, regulation of prostitution, sexual exploitation of children, Internet porn, gays and lesbians in the military, gay 'marriage' and adoption, hate crimes, new reproductive technologies, and the 'private' morality of politicians are the topic of intense public debate, and older issues such as access to abortion are currently subjected to renewed contestation. Issues such as Aids, sex tourism, international trafficking of women, and Internet networks of paedophiles illustrate the global nature of politics of sexuality, as well as the resurgence of moral purity discourses and their political influence. Against the backdrop of the politics of sexuality, as well as wider social and technological developments, sexuality has undergone profound changes over the past few decades. Modern sexual science has

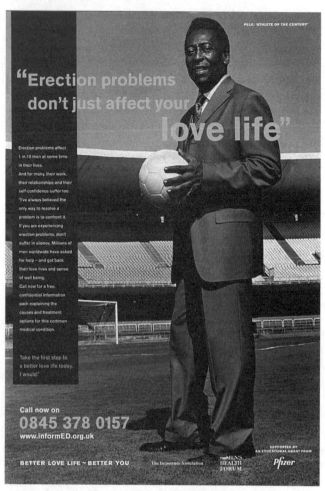

13. Pfizer/The Impotence Association magazine advertisement, featuring the football legend Pelé, which appeared in 2002

documented the impact of such changes on individual practices. Somewhat ironically, the primary agents in the transformation of sexual truths and relations of power are those that medicine and sexology had constructed as marginal in relation to hegemonic male heterosexuality, namely women and homosexuals of both sexes, as we have seen throughout this volume.

In the process, social understandings of sexuality have opened up to a plurality of meanings. Whereas liberation theorists saw sexual pleasure as crucial for the fulfilment of full human potential and happiness, competing understandings have portrayed sexuality as the site of risk, death, moral decay, commercial exploitation, male violence, political self-affirmation, and destabilization of identities.

Liquid sex

Modern individuals can in principle adopt sexual identities at will, but they do not do so in conditions of their own choosing. The social and political context of modernity sets the stage for sexual possibilities. For example, new communication technologies such as the Internet provide new sexual options, including the adoption of 'virtual' identities in cyberspace as well as greater access to potential partners. The modern world, as the sociologist Zygmunt Bauman argues in his book *Liquid Love*, is characterized by fluidity in social relations generally, encouraging a reluctance towards long-term commitments since a 'better product' might be just around the corner. The fragmentation of sexual subcultures is mirrored in the specialization of the commodities on offer. Gay men's dating websites such as Gaydar have become global phenomena, with users including men from countries such as Algeria, Afghanistan, Pakistan, or the Democratic Republic of Congo. More specialized dating agencies cater for 'heterosexual, gentile (non-Jewish), whites only', 'gay black females', or the 'unhappily married/attached', while the now defunct Safe Love International, which included prominent sexologists such as

Theresa Crenshaw on its advisory council, promised that its members were 'Aids-free'.

Citizens of the modern sexual world make sense of their personal identities and problems in new ways, as reflected in a recent dilemma submitted to the popular internationally syndicated Internet relationship and sex advice column 'Savage Love', run by American gay author of *Skipping Towards Gomorrah* (2002) Dan Savage:

> For the past 15 years, I've identified as bisexual: I've been in monogamous relationships with men and women. I married a wonderful guy a few years ago. However, I recently realised that I identify as gay. I've talked to my husband about this, and he's okay with it. I decided to stay with him and remain monogamous. We have a great relationship – and great sex. We left open the possibility of me taking a female lover in the future, if needed. For now, I'm happy with him. I flirt with girls, we talk openly about my preferences, but I haven't had sex with a woman since before I married him. And I'm okay with that. So, here's my dilemma: Is it right to call myself a lesbian if I'm married to (and sexually involved with) a man? I hesitate to stay with the 'bi' label, since I have no interest in other men. Can I call myself a lesbian even though I'm not sleeping with women?

Advice columns, agony aunts, therapists, support groups such as Sex Addicts Anonymous, self-help books, and sex manuals can be drawn upon to offer advice on relationship rules, sexual etiquette, and sexual mechanics in the liquid world of modern sex. Titles such as *Women Who Love Too Much*, *Relationship Rescue*, *How to Fall Out of Love*, or *If It Hurts, It Isn't Love* guide readers through the minefield of intimacy and emotions. Other works privilege a more practical angle, such as *Sexercise* ('will help you get fit while you're having fun!'), *This Book Will Get You Laid* ('the bonking bible no bloke should be without'), or American sexologist Dr Ruth's *Sex for Dummies*. Specific subgroups are catered for by works such as *The Adventurous Couple's Guide to Strap-On Sex*, *The Gay Joy of Sex*, *Sex: A Man's Guide*, *The New Love and Sex After 60*, *The Lesbian Sex Book*, or *Enabling Romance: A Guide to Love, Sex and Relationships for People with Disabilities (and for the People Who Care About Them)*.

Best-selling self-help books such as *The Rules: Time-Tested Secrets for Capturing the Heart of Mr. Right* (1995) reproduce traditional norms of female and male sexual behaviour and needs, based upon the claim that men and women are biologically different creatures. 'In a relationship, the man must take charge. He must propose. We are not making this up – biologically, he's the aggressor', as the *Rules*, such as 'don't talk to a man first (and don't ask him to dance)', formulate it.

Attempts to break away from dominant norms frequently involve the formulation of new normativities, however, as illustrated by Shere Hite's emphasis on the necessity for women to experience sexual pleasure:

> If you can't orgasm, you could also read books on sex therapy, feminist literature, and try to talk to friends about how they have orgasms. You could also try a local women's self-help group, perhaps a sex-therapist, or a lover who was sensitive enough to help. *Don't give up*. Many women *have* learned to orgasm after years of not knowing how, and it is never too late to discover what works for *you*.

The current transformations and politics of sexuality have started to problematize the hegemony as well as the forms of 'normality'. Feminist critiques of sexuality have encouraged wider understandings of sexuality, less centred on penetrative intercourse alone, while gay and lesbian communities of choice and attendant political activism have publicly demonstrated the profound transformations of both the sexual order and the gender order of the West in recent decades.

In their radical experiments with intersections between gender and sexuality, the 'queers' queers' are perhaps the sexual revolutionaries of our time. Just as self-castrating early Christians, anarchist free-lovers, 1960s swingers, Reichian sexual liberationists, and political lesbians came from the periphery of the continent of sex to invent new meanings and practices, so the pomosexual 'lesbian separatist who becomes a professional dominatrix, then falls in love with a male-to-female transsexual grrl, decides to go through with a sex change, becomes a guy, and realizes he's a gay man' questions our most basic assumptions about gender and sexual identity, and illustrates the possibilities for greater fluidity that the (post)modern world offers.

Does that mean that, in future, we will all think of ourselves as pomosexuals? Are we currently witnessing the final death throes of heterosexuality and homosexuality? As we have seen, current sexual 'truths' and identities are relatively recent historical constructs, produced by sexual science and medicine. The future of sex may well involve leaving behind the constraints of 19th-century 'sexuality'. Theorists of sexuality have thus called for collective 'un-sexualization'. At the same time, there is little in the current state of the politics of sexuality to lead us to conclude that an 'unsexual' future is anywhere near, given the renewed propping up of traditional understandings of sex by the fundamentalist backlash, as well as by scientific discourses. What is certain, however, is that alternative futures of sex based on moral pluralism cannot escape new normativities, new relations of power, and new state policies. No culture can have 'full' sexual freedom. As the sociologist Ken Plummer puts it:

> However neutral and objective talk about sexual diversity appears to be, it is also talk about power. Every culture has to establish – through both formal and informal political processes – the range and scope of the diversities that will be outlawed or banned.

As this volume has argued, sexual needs, values, and emotions are the products of specific historical contexts. Current practices may contribute to undermining concepts of 'sexuality', but, whatever changes scientific and technological developments will bring to our bodies and relationships, future meanings of sex will be shaped by society and politics.

References and further reading

Chapter 1

For an authoritative analysis of sex in the Greek literature of the first centuries AD: Simon Goldhill, *Foucault's Virginity: Ancient Erotic Fiction and the History of Sexuality* (Cambridge: Cambridge University Press, 1995). The title quote is from *Erotes* 36 and cited in Goldhill's book, p. ix.

For Plato's *Symposium*, the established Loeb edition, with English translation added, is recommended: Plato, *Volume III*, Loeb Classical Library (Harvard: Harvard University Press, 1925).

For Ovid's *Metamorphoses* (myth of Tiresias), *Ars Amatoria* and *Remedia Amoris*: *Ovid, Volumes III, IV, and II*, Loeb Classical Library (Harvard: Harvard University Press, revised edn 1979).

The quotation from Demosthenes is from *Oration* 59.122.

The quotes from Petronius's *Satyricon* (Loeb Classical Library, Harvard: Harvard University Press, revised edn 1969), and from Priscianus (2.11), are borrowed from Angus McLaren, *Impotence: A Cultural History* (Chicago: Chicago University Press, 2007), pp. 2 and 15.

For Michel Foucault's analyses of sex in antiquity: see his two volumes *The History of Sexuality, Volume II: The Use of Pleasure* (New York: Random House, 1985 [1984]) and *The History of Sexuality, Volume III: The Care of the Self* (New York: Random House, 1986 [1984]). David Halperin's writings offer influential accounts of sex in ancient Greece, in a broadly Foucauldian perspective: see, in particular, his *One Hundred Years of Homosexuality and Other Essays on Greek Love* (New York: Routledge, 1990); Halperin's quotation on citizenship is on p. 11 of this work. A similar perspective is developed in John J. Winkler, *The Constraints of Desire: The Anthropology of Sex and Gender in Ancient Greece* (New York: Routledge, 1990).

For contrasting analyses: John Boswell's controversial *Same-Sex Unions in Premodern Europe* (New York: Random House, 1994); and James Davidson, *Courtesans and Fishcakes: The Consuming Passions of Classical Athens* (London: Fontana Press, 1998), which discusses sex, food, and drink – his quote on 'managing all appetites' is from p. 313. On the links between food and sex, see also Peter Garnsey, *Food and Society in Classical Antiquity* (Cambridge: Cambridge University Press, 1999).

On female sexuality and the body in antiquity: Helen King, *Hippocrates's Woman: Reading the Female Body in Ancient Greece* (London: Routledge, 1998); and Sarah B. Pomeroy, *Goddesses, Whores, Wives and Slaves: Women in Classical Antiquity* (New York: Schocken Books, 1975); see also Rebecca Flemming, *Medicine and the Making of Roman Women: Gender, Nature, and Authority from Celsus to Galen* (Oxford: Oxford University Press, 2000) on ancient medicine.

On the term 'lesbiazein': James Clackson and Simon Goldhill, personal communication. See also Jeffrey Henderson, *The Maculate Muse: Obscene Language in Attic Comedy*, 2nd edn (Oxford: Oxford University Press, 1991), p. 183.

Seneca's quotation on morality and perversity is from *De Beneficiis*, 1.10. The comment to Lucilius is from Seneca, *Letter* 97.

Pliny's discussion of elephant love: Pliny, *Natural History* 8.5, Loeb Classical Library (Volume 3) (Harvard: Harvard University Press, 1942).

For a respected guide to early Christian views on sex: Peter Brown, *The Body and Society: Men, Women and Sexual Renunciation in Early Christianity* (New York: Columbia Press, 1988).

The examination for impotence is reported in Angus McLaren, *Impotence: A Cultural History* (Chicago: Chicago University Press, 2007), and originally quoted in Richard H. Helmholtz, *Marriage Litigation in Medieval England* (Cambridge: Cambridge University Press, 1974), p. 89.

On Origen and self-castration: Uta Ranke-Heinemann, *Eunuchs for Heaven: The Catholic Church and Sexuality*, tr. John Brownjohn (London: Deutsch, 1990).

For Augustine's views: *The Confessions of St. Augustine*, ed. James O'Donnell (Oxford: Clarendon Press, 1992) and his *Letters*, especially *On the Good of Marriage*.

On sex, gender, and the body: Thomas Laqueur, *Making Sex: Body and Gender from the Greeks to Freud* (Harvard: Harvard University Press, 1990).

On Florence's Office of the Night: Michael Rocke, *Forbidden Friendships: Homosexuality and Male Culture in Renaissance Florence* (Oxford: Oxford University Press, 1996).

Chapter 2

The title quote is from Richard von Krafft-Ebing, *Psychopathia Sexualis* (New York: Arcade Publishing, 1998 [1886]), pp. 263–4.

Foucault's views on sexuality: Michel Foucault, *The History of Sexuality, Volume I: An Introduction* (Harmondsworth: Penguin, 1990 [1976]). The quotation on 'the sodomite' is on p. 43; his quote on 'the confessing society' is on p. 59. See also Véronique Mottier, 'Sexuality and Sexology: Michel Foucault', pp. 113–23 in Terrell Carver and Véronique Mottier (eds), *Politics of Sexuality: Identity, Gender, Citizenship* (London: Routledge, 1998).

Excellent historical overviews: Stephen Garton, *Histories of Sexuality: Antiquity to Sexual Revolution* (London: Equinox, 2004). On the UK specifically, see Jeffrey Weeks, *Sex, Politics and Society: The Regulation of Sexuality since 1800*, 2nd edn (Harlow: Longman, 1998) – the quote on sexology as a continent of knowledge is on p. 142, the quote on 'sex reformers' is on p. 145; and Steven Marcus, *The Other Victorians: A Study of Sexuality and Pornography in Mid-Nineteenth-Century England* (New York: Basic Books, 1964).

Masturbation: Thomas Laqueur, *Solitary Sex: A Cultural History of Masturbation* (New York: Zone Books, 2003); Anonymous, *Onania; or, the Heinous Sin of Self Pollution, and all its Frightful Consequences, in both SEXES considered, with Spiritual and Physical Advice to those who have already injured themselves by this abominable Practice* (London, appr. 1712/1718); Samuel Tissot, *L'Onanisme; ou, Dissertation physique sur les maladies produites par la masturbation* (Paris, 1760).

The quotation on the volcanic element of sex is from Patrick Geddes and J. A. Thomson, *Sex* (London: Home Universal Library, 1914), p. 148.

On the coining of sexual categories: Jonathan Ned Katz, *The Invention of Heterosexuality* (Chicago: University of Chicago Press, 2007); Katz's quotation on 'sex history's grand ironies' is on p. 53. Joséphin Péladan, *Le vice supreme* (Lyon: Editions Palimpseste, 2006 [1884]). Also Volume I of Foucault's *History of Sexuality* and the *Oxford English Dictionary*.

For excerpts from many classic works in early sexology, see Lucy Bland and Laura Doan (eds), *Sexology Uncensored: The Documents of Sexual Science* (Cambridge: Polity Press, 1998).

The 'one-sex body': Thomas Laqueur, *Making Sex: Body and Gender from the Greeks to Freud* (Harvard: Harvard University Press, 1990). The quote from William Acton is cited in this work, p. 190.

On 19th-century clitoridectomy: Helen King, *Hippocrates's Woman: Reading the Female Body in Ancient Greece* (London: Routledge, 1998), p. 14.

Famous early erotic novels: John Cleland, *Fanny Hill: or Memoirs of a Woman of Pleasure* (London: Wordsworth Editions, 2000 [1748–9]); 'Walter' (Anonymous), *My Secret Life* (London: Wordsworth Editions, 1995 [1888–94]).

Quotes from Forel are from: Auguste Forel, *The Sexual Question* (London: Heinemann, 1908 [1906]).

'Coital orgasmic inadequacy': William Masters and Virginia Johnson, *Human Sexual Inadequacy* (Boston, Mass.: Little Brown, 1970).

German 19th-century movements for the rights of homosexuals: Eve Kosofsky Sedgwick, *Epistemology of the Closet* (Berkeley: University of California Press, 1990), pp. 88 and 134.

Sexual liberation theorists: Wilhelm Reich, *The Sexual Revolution: Toward a Self-Governing Character Structure*, 4th edn (New York: Farrar, Straus and Giroux, 1969 [1930]). His quotes on sexuality as 'the life energy *per se*', 'authoritarian social order', and 'orgasm anxiety' are from this book, pp. xxv, xxix, and 448. Reich's quotations on 'neurotic patients', 'sex-economist' and 'orgastic potency' are from his 1948 text 'The Orgasm Theory', pp. 37, 42, and 43 in *Selected Writings: An Introduction to Orgonomy* (New York: Farrar, Straus and Giroux, 1960). Herbert Marcuse, *Eros and Civilisation:*

A Philosophical Inquiry into Freud (London: Routledge, 1956); Erich Fromm, *The Art of Loving* (London: Continuum, 2000 [1956]).

Sex surveys: Vern L. Bullough, *Science in the Bedroom: The History of Sex Research* (New York: Basic Books, 1994); Liz Stanley, *Sex Surveyed 1949-1994* (London: Taylor & Francis, 1995).

The Kinsey Reports: Alfred C. Kinsey et al., *Sexual Behaviour in the Human Male* (Philadelphia: Saunders, 1949); *Sexual Behaviour in the Human Female* (Philadelphia: Saunders, 1953).

Masters and Johnson: William Masters and Virginia Johnson, *Human Sexual Response* (New York: Bantam Books, 1966); *Human Sexual Inadequacy* (Boston, Mass.: Little Brown, 1970).

Freud: Sigmund Freud, *Civilisation and Its Discontents*, tr. James Strachey (New York: Norton, 1989 [1915]); *Three Essays on the Theory of Sexuality* (New York: Basic Books, 2000 [1905]). See also Juliet Mitchell, *Psychoanalysis and Feminism: Freud, Reich, Laing, and Women* (New York: Pantheon Books, 1974); Mitchell's quote 'in childhood all is diverse or perverse' is on p. 19.

Recent examples of evolutionary perspectives on sexuality: Randy Thornhill and Craig Palmer, *A Natural History of Rape: Biological Bases of Sexual Coercion* (Cambridge, Mass.: MIT Press, 2000); Michael P. Ghiglieri, *The Dark Side of Man: Tracing the Origins of Male Violence* (New York: Perseus, 1999); Helen Fischer, *Anatomy of Love: A Natural History of Mating, Marriage, and Why We Stray* (New York: Random House, 1992).

Key works developing social models of sexuality – in sociology: John H. Gagnon and W. Simon, *Sexual Conduct: The Social Sources of Human Sexuality* (Chicago: Aldine, 1973); Ken Plummer, *Sexual Stigma: An Interactionist Account* (London: Routledge & Kegan Paul, 1975); Jeffrey Weeks, *Sexuality and Its Discontents: Meanings,*

Myths and Modern Sexualities (London: Routledge & Kegan Paul, 1985); Weeks's quote on 'the speaking perverts' is on p. 21; – in literary criticism: Stephen Heath, *The Sexual Fix* (Houndmills: MacMillan, 1982); – in classics: David Halperin, *One Hundred Years of Homosexuality and Other Essays on Greek Love* (New York: Routledge, 1990).

Chapter 3

The title quote is from Jill Johnson, *Lesbian Nation* (New York: Simon and Schuster, 1973), pp. 166–7.

Syphilis/venereal disease: Tamsin Wilton, *EnGendering AIDS: Deconstructing Sex, Text and Epidemic* (London: Sage, 1997); the quote from Shakespeare's *King Lear*, Act IV. v 126, is cited on p. 59, the slogan 'VD worst of the three' on p. 62. Derek Llewellyn-Jones, *Herpes, AIDS and Other Sexually Transmitted Diseases* (London: Faber and Faber, 1985); the quote on 'the Spanish disease' is on p. 136. Magnus Hirschfeld, *The Sexual History of the World War* (Honolulu: University Press of the Pacific, 2006 [1941]).

Policies and feminist activism around prostitution: Lucy Bland, *Banishing the Beast: English Feminism and Sexual Morality 1885–1914* (London: Penguin, 1995); William Acton's outburst on female insubordination is cited on p. 55, the 'Women Against Sex' quotation is on p. 313. Philippa Levine, *Prostitution, Race and Politics: Policing Venereal Disease in the British Empire* (New York: Routledge, 2003). Joyce Outshoorn (ed.), *The Politics of Prostitution: Women's Movements, Democratic States and the Globalisation of Sex Commerce* (Cambridge: Cambridge University Press, 2004) discusses current prostitution policies across the world.

Kollontai's views: Alexandra Kollontai, 'Communism and the Family', first published in *Kommunistka*, no. 2 (1920); 'Theses on Communist Morality in the Sphere of Marital Relations', first published in *Kommunistka*, no. 12 (1921).

Giddens's quote on a revolution in 'female sexual autonomy' is from Anthony Giddens, *The Transformation of Intimacy: Sexuality, Love and Eroticism in Modern Societies* (Cambridge: Polity Press, 1992), p. 29.

Masturbation: Betty Dodson, *Liberating Masturbation: A Meditation on Self-Loving* (Bodysex Designs, 1974) and *Sex For One* (New York: Three Rivers Press, 1986); see also Dodson's recent DVD, 'Selfloving: Video Portrait of a Women's Sexuality Seminar'.

Alex Comfort, *The Joy of Sex* (New York: Crown, 1972 and various later revised editions); *More Joy of Sex* (London: Mitchell Beazley, 1973 and various later revised editions).

Feminist views on the sexual revolution: Sheila Jeffreys, *Anticlimax: A Feminist Perspective on the Sexual Revolution* (London: The Women's Press, 1990). Beatrix Campbell, 'A Feminist Sexual Politics: Now You See It Now You Don't', *Feminist Review*, 5 (1980): 1–18; her quote on 'the permissive era' is on pp. 1–2. Kate Millett, *Sexual Politics* (London: Virago, 1970). Germaine Greer, *Female Eunuch* (New York: Farrar, Straus and Giroux, 1971).

Masters and Johnson and women's liberation (in sex): William Masters and Virginia Johnson, *The Pleasure Bond* (New York: Bantam Books, 1974). For a critical analysis, see Janice M. Irvine, *Disorders of Desire: Sex and Gender in Modern American Sexology* (Philadelphia: Temple University Press, 1990).

Friday's famous studies of sexual fantasies: Nancy Friday, *My Secret Garden: Women's Sexual Fantasies* (New York: Pocket Books, 1973); *Forbidden Flowers: More Women's Sexual Fantasies* (New York: Pocket Books, 1975); *Men in Love: Men's Sexual Fantasies; The Triumph of Love over Rage* (New York: Dell, 1980).

Female orgasm/frigidity: Frank Caprio, *The Sexually Adequate Woman* (New York: The Citadel Press, 1963); his quote is on p. 64.

Marie Bonaparte, *Female Sexuality* (New York: Grove Press, 1953).
Anne Koedt, 'The Myth of the Vaginal Orgasm', in her *Radical Feminism* (New York: Quadrangle, 1972). Alix Shulman, 'Organs and Orgasms', in *Women in Sexist Society: Studies in Power and Powerlessness*, ed. Vivian Gornick and Barbara K. Moran (New York: Signet Books, 1972), p. 296; also cited in *The Hite Report on Female Sexuality*, p. 275.

The Hite Reports: Shere Hite, *The Hite Report on Female Sexuality* (New York: Dell, 1976). Her quote on 'lack of sexual satisfaction' is on p. 420; her quote on '95 percent could orgasm' is on p. 59; her quote 'the fact that women can orgasm easily' is on p. 60; her quote on 'sexual slavery' is on p. 419. Shere Hite, *The Hite Report on Male Sexuality* (New York: Ballantine, 1981); her quote on 'rape' is on p. 742. Véronique Mottier, 'The Politics of Sex: Truth Games and the Hite Reports', *Economy and Society*, 24, 4 (1995): 520–39.

Political lesbianism: Leeds Revolutionary Feminist Group, *Love Thy Enemy? The Debate between Heterosexual Feminism and Political Lesbianism* (London: Onlywomenpress, 1981). Adrienne Rich, 'Compulsory Heterosexuality and Lesbian Existence', *Signs*, 5, 4 (1980): 631–60. Radicalesbians, 'The Woman-Identified Woman', conference pamphlet 1970. 'Editorial', *Nouvelles Questions Féministes*, 1 March 1981; the quotes 'all women are oppressed', 'terrorist', and 'totalitarian' are on pp. 6–7 (my translation).

Sexual violence: Susan Brownmiller, *Against Our Will: Men, Women, and Rape* (London: Secker & Warburg, 1975). Andrea Dworkin, *Intercourse* (New York: Simon & Schuster, 1997 [1987]); the quote 'in the fuck' is on p. 66. Susan Griffin, *Pornography and Silence* (New York: Harper & Row, 1981). For contrasting views on masculinity and sex: Lynne Segal, *Slow Motion; Changing Masculinities, Changing Men* (London: Virago, revised edn 1997); her quote 'for many men' is on p. 212.

Feminist sex wars: Lisa Duggan and Nan D. Hunter, *Sex Wars: Sexual Dissent and Political Culture* (New York: Routledge, 1995).

Female genital mutilation: Gloria Steinem and Robin Morgan, 'The International Crime of Genital Mutilation', in *Outrageous Acts and Everyday Rebellions*, ed. Gloria Steinem (New York: Holt, Rinehart, and Winston, 1983), pp. 292–8. Alice Walker, *Possessing the Secret of Joy* (London: Jonathan Cape, 1992). Alice Walker and Pratibha Parmar, *Warrior Marks: Female Genital Mutilation and the Sexual Blinding of Women* (San Diego: Harvest, 1993). Nontsasa Nako, 'Possessing the Voice of the Other: African Women and the "Crisis of Representation" in Alice Walker's Possessing the Secret of Joy', *Jenda – A Journal of Culture and African Women's Studies*, 1, 2 (2001).

Chapter 4

The title quote is from Angela Franks, *Margaret Sanger's Eugenic Legacy: The Control of Female Fertility* (Jefferson: McFarland, 2005), p. 34. Sanger's quotes 'nature eliminates the weeds' and 'clog up the path' are on p. 48; the *Buck vs Bell* decision is on p. 183.

'The sexual revolution was heterosexual': the quote is from Sheila Jeffreys, *Anticlimax: A Feminist Perspective on the Sexual Revolution* (London: The Women's Press, 1990), p. 110.

Aids and the (unfinished) sexual revolution: Jeffrey Weeks, *Sex, Politics and Society: The Regulation of Sexuality since 1800*, 2nd edn (Harlow: Longman, 1998), p. 302; the Chief Constable of Manchester's quote is on p. 301; the quote 'the impact of the Aids crisis' is on p. 304.

American sexology and responses to Aids: Janice M. Irvine, *Disorders of Desire: Sex and Gender in Modern American Sexology* (Philadelphia: Temple University Press, 1990); Crenshaw's quote 'the sexual revolution is over' is cited on p. 153. William Masters, Virginia Johnson, and Robert Kolodny, *Crisis: Heterosexual Behavior in the Age of Aids* (New York: Grove Press, 1988).

Feminist research on Aids: Janet Holland, Caroline Ramazanoglu, Rachel Thomson, and Sue Sharpe, *The Male in the Head: Young People, Heterosexuality and Power* (London: The Tufnell Press, 1998).

Michel Foucault, 'Non au sexe roi', in *Dits et ecrits 1954–1988 par Michel Foucault*, vol. 3, ed. Daniel Defert and François Ewald (Paris: Gallimard, 2004), pp. 256–69; the quote 'sexuality has always been' is on p. 257.

Auguste Forel's quotes 'the regulation of procreation', 'let science enlighten', and 'each fiancée has the right' are from his pamphlet *Le rôle de l'hypocrisie, de la bêtise et de l'ignorance dans la morale contemporaine* (Lausanne: Libre Pensée Internationale, 1916); his quote 'an intelligent, scientific social-democracy' is from his pamphlet *La morale en soi* (Lausanne: Administration de la libre pensée, 1910), my translation.

Eugenics in Switzerland: Véronique Mottier and Laura von Mandach (eds), *Eugenik und Disziplinierung in der Schweiz: Integration und Ausschluss in Psychiatrie, Medizin und Fürsorge* (Zurich: Seismo, 2007); this edited volume presents summaries of recent archival research by Swiss historians Regina Wecker, Jakob Tanner, Roswitha Dubach, Marietta Meier, Beatrice Ziegler, Gisela Hauss, and their research teams. See also: Véronique Mottier, 'Eugenics and the Swiss Gender Regime: Women's Bodies and the Struggle against "Difference"', *Revue Suisse de Sociologie*, 32, 1 (2006): 253–67; Natalia Gerodetti, 'From Science to Social Technology: Eugenics and Politics in Twentieth-Century Switzerland', *Social Politics: International Studies in Gender, State and Society*, 13, 1 (2006): 59–88 and 'Eugenic Family Politics and Social Democrats: "Positive" Eugenics and Marriage Advice Bureaus', *Journal of Historical Sociology*, 19, 3 (2006): 217–44; Gilles Jeanmonod and Geneviève Heller, 'Eugénisme et contexte socio-politique: l'exemple de l'adoption d'une loi sur la stérilisation des handicapés et malades mentaux dans le canton de Vaud en 1928', *Revue d'histoire suisse*, 50 (2000): 20–44.

Eugenics in Scandinavia: Gunnar Broberg and Nils Roll-Hansen, *Eugenics and the Welfare State: Norway, Sweden, Denmark, and Finland* (Michigan: Michigan State University Press, 2005).

Eugenics and the Left: Diane Paul, 'Eugenics and the Left', *Journal of the History of Ideas*, 45, 4 (1984): 567–90; Véronique Mottier and Natalia Gerodetti, 'Eugenics and Social-Democracy: or, How the Left Tried to Eliminate the "Weeds" from its National Gardens', *New Formations*, 60 (2007): 35–49.

Eugenics in the United States: Wendy Kline, *Building a Better Race: Gender, Sexuality and Eugenics from the Turn of the Century to the Baby Boom* (Berkeley: University of California Press, 2001).

Female sexuality and nationalism: Nira Yuval-Davis, *Gender and Nation* (London: Sage, 1997).

Swiss child removal programme: Walter Leimgruber, Thomas Meier, and Roger Sablonier, *Das Hilfswerk fuer die Kinder der Landstrasse* (Bern: Schweiz. Bundesarchiv, 1998).

Hirschfeld's quote 'an interesting experiment': Magnus Hirschfeld, *Racism* (London: Gollanz, 1938).

Chapter 5

The title quote is from Jeffrey Weeks, *Sexuality* (London: Routledge), p. 77. His quote 'a great continent of normality' is on p. 80.

'Like their male counterparts': the quote is from David Reuben, *Everything You Ever Wanted to Know About Sex But Was Afraid to Ask* (London: W. H. Allen, 1970), p. 215.

Debates around 'gay marriage': see Claire R. Snyder, *Gay Marriage and Democracy: Equality for All* (Lanham: Rowman & Littlefield, 2006).

Age of consent battles: see Matthew Waites, *The Age of Consent: Young People, Sexuality and Citizenship* (New York: Palgrave MacMillan, 2005).

'they are not part of our community': the quote is from gay rights activist Gregory King, cited in Joshua Gamson, 'Messages of Exclusion: Gender, Movements, and Symbolic Boundaries', *Gender and Society*, 11, 2 (1997): 178–99.

Gay vs gender separatism: see Eve Kosofski Sedgwick, *Epistemology of the Closet* (Berkeley: University of California Press, 1990), pp. 88–90; Jill Johnson, *Lesbian Nation* (New York: Simon & Schuster, 1973).

Tales of the City series: this refers to a series of six novels, the first titled *Tales of the City*, written by Armistead Maupin and published between 1978 and 1990, chronicling the lives of various main characters in San Francisco.

Neo-pagan feminism: Zsuzanna Budapest, *The Holy Book of Women's Mysteries* (Oakland, California: Wingbow Publishers, 1989), originally published under a different title in 1975.

'We are … past such identities': the quote is from Diana Richardson, *Rethinking Sexuality* (London: Sage, 2000), pp. 38–9.

'In a nutshell': the quote is from Carol Queen and Lawrence Schimel (eds), *PoMoSexuals: Challenging Assumptions about Gender and Sexuality* (San Francisco: Cleis Press, 1997), pp. 13–14; the quotation 'We pomosexuals are the queer's queers' is on pp. 24–5; the quote from Travers Scott, 'Queer almost immediately came to mean …' is on p. 64; Pat Califia's quote on PoMoSexuals as the 'bastard children' is on p. 103; 'lesbian separatist who becomes a professional dominatrix' is on p. 16.

'Progressive' sexual value models: Jeffrey Weeks, *Invented Moralities: Sexual Values in an Age of Uncertainty* (Cambridge: Polity Press, 1995).

Andrew Sullivan, *The Conservative Soul: How We Lost It, How to Get It Back* (New York: Harper Collins, 2006).

Sexuality and 'race': Edward W. Said, *Orientalism* (London: Routledge & Kegan Paul, 1978); Margaret Mead, *Coming of Age in Samoa: A Psychological Study of Primitive Youth for Western Civilization* (New York: Perennial, 2001 [1928]); Bronislaw Malinowski, *The Sexual Life of Savages* (Boston: Beacon Press, 1987 [1929]).

Sexuality as 'an especially dense transfer point': the quotation is from Michel Foucault, *The History of Sexuality, Volume I: An Introduction* (Harmondsworth: Penguin, 1990 [1976]), p. 103.

Sexuality as 'a malleable feature of self': the quotation is from Anthony Giddens, *The Transformation of Intimacy: Sexuality, Love and Eroticism in Modern Societies* (Cambridge: Polity Press, 1992), p. 15.

'men's liberation is a passive affair': the quotation is from Ulrich Beck and Elizabeth Beck-Gernsheim, *The Normal Chaos of Love* (Cambridge: Polity Press, 1995), p. 153.

'Gender is not a synonym for women': book-title of Terrell Carver, *Gender is Not a Synonym for Women* (Boulder, Colorado: Lynne Rienner, 1996).

'Liquid love': Zygmunt Bauman, *Liquid Love: On the Frailty of Human Bonds* (Cambridge: Polity Press, 2003).

Advice literature: the quotation 'for the past 15 years ...' is from Dan Savage's advice column of 7 November 2007. See also Dan Savage, *Skipping Towards Gomorrah: The Seven Deadly Sins and the Pursuit of Happiness in America* (New York: Plume, 2002). The quotation 'the man must take charge' is from *The Complete Book of Rules: Time-Tested Secrets for Capturing the Heart of Mr. Right* (London: Harper Collins, 2000), p. 7; this is an expanded edition of the original 1995 work *The Rules*.

'If you can't orgasm': the quote is from Shere Hite, *The Hite Report on Female Sexuality* (New York: Dell, 1976), p. 222.

Sexual diversity and power: the quote 'however neutral and objective ...' is from Ken Plummer, 'Sexual Diversity: A Sociological Perspective', in *Sexual Diversity*, ed. Kevin Howells (Oxford: Blackwell, 1984), p. 219.

The politics of sex: see Terrell Carver and Véronique Mottier (eds), *Politics of Sexuality: Identity, Gender, Citizenship* (London: Routledge, 1998).

Index

Index

Sexuality

Sexuality

SOCIOLOGY
A Very Short Introduction
Steve Bruce

Drawing on studies of social class, crime and deviance, work in bureaucracies, and changes in religious and political organizations, this Very Short Introduction explores the tension between the individual's role in society and society's role in shaping the individual, and demonstrates the value of sociology as a perspective for understanding the modern world.

'Steve Bruce has made an excellent job of a difficult task, one which few practising sociologists could have accomplished with such aplomb. The arguments are provocatively and intelligently presented, and the tone and the style are also laudable.'

Gordon Marshall, University of Oxford

FREUD
A Very Short Introduction
Anthony Storr

Sigmund Freud revolutionised the way in which we think
about ourselves. From its beginnings as a theory of
neurosis, Freud developed psychoanalysis into a general
psychology which became widely accepted as the
predominant mode of discussing personality and
interpersonal relationships. Anthony Storr goes one step
further and investigates the status of Freud's legacy today
and the disputes that surround it.

> 'lucid, fair and astonishingly comprehensive . . . A useful
> and illuminating little book.'
>
> **Spectator**

> 'brief, elegant and interesting'
>
> **D.M. Thomas, *Observer***

> 'A lucid, unbiased account which will help to put Freudian
> theory into proper perspective'
>
> **D. Roger, University of York**

www.oup.co.uk/isbn/0-19-285455-0

SOCIAL AND CULTURAL ANTHROPOLOGY
A Very Short Introduction

John Monaghan and Peter Just

'If you want to know what anthropology *is*, look at what anthropologists *do*.'

This Very Short Introduction to Social and Cultural Anthropology combines an accessible account of some of the discipline's guiding principles and methodology with abundant examples and illustrations of anthropologists at work.

Peter Just and John Monaghan begin by discussing anthropology's most important contributions to modern thought: its investigation of culture as a distinctly 'human' characteristic, its doctrine of cultural relativism, and its methodology of fieldwork and ethnography. They then examine specific ways in which social and cultural anthropology have advanced our understanding of human society and culture, drawing on examples from their own fieldwork. The book ends with an assessment of anthropology's present position, and a look forward to its likely future.

www.oup.co.uk/vsi/anthropology

THE MARQUIS DE SADE

A Very Short Introduction

John Phillips

Were it not for the Marquis de Sade's explicit use of language and complete disregard for the artificially constructed taboos of a religious morality he despised, the novelty and profundity of his thought, and above all, its fundamental modernity, would have long since secured him a place alongside the greatest authors and thinkers of the European Enlightenment.

This Very Short Introduction aims to disentangle the 'real' Marquis de Sade from his mythical and demonic reputation of the past two hundred years. Phillips examines Sade's life and work: his libertine novels, his championing of atheism, and his uniqueness in bringing the body and sex back into philosophy.

http://www.oup.co.uk/isbn/0–19–280469–3

MYTH
A Very Short Introduction
Robert A. Segal

This book is not about myths, but about approaches to myth, from all of the major disciplines, including science, religion, philosophy, literature, and psychology. Segal uses the fable of beautiful Adonis in an attempt to analyse the various different theories of myth. Where the theory does not work, he substitutes another myth, showing that, certain theories, in fact, only apply to specific kinds of myths.

A survey of the past 300 years of theorizing on myth, this book takes into account the work of such prominent thinkers as Albert Camus, Claude Lévi-Strauss, Roland Barthes, C. G. Jung, and Sigmund Freud. Finally, Segal considers the future study of myth, and the possible function of myth in the world as the adult equivalent of play.

'Segal's writing is entirely lucid'
Laurence Phelan, Independent on Sunday

http://www.oup.co.uk/isbn/0-19-280347-6